MYTHS OF TRAUMA

MYTHS OF TRAUMA

Why Adversity Does Not Necessarily Make Us Sick

Joel Paris

PROFESSOR EMERITUS OF PSYCHIATRY, MCGILL UNIVERSITY

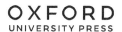

OXFORD
UNIVERSITY PRESS

Oxford University Press is a department of the University of Oxford. It furthers
the University's objective of excellence in research, scholarship, and education
by publishing worldwide. Oxford is a registered trade mark of Oxford University
Press in the UK and certain other countries.

Published in the United States of America by Oxford University Press
198 Madison Avenue, New York, NY 10016, United States of America.

Library of Congress Cataloging-in-Publication Data
Names: Paris, Joel, 1940– author.
Title: Myths of trauma : why adversity does not
necessarily make us sick / Joel Paris.
Description: New York, NY : Oxford University Press, [2023] |
Includes bibliographical references and index. |
Identifiers: LCCN 2022010908 (print) | LCCN 2022010909 (ebook) |
ISBN 9780197615768 (paperback) | ISBN 9780197615782 (epub) |
ISBN 9780197615799 (online)
Subjects: MESH: Diagnostic and statistical manual of mental disorders. 5th ed. |
Psychological Trauma | Stress Disorders, Post-Traumatic—etiology |
Mental Disorders—diagnosis | Risk Assessment | Resilience, Psychological
Classification: LCC RC552.T7 (print) | LCC RC552.T7 (ebook) |
NLM WM 172.5 | DDC 616.85/21—dc23/eng/20220323
LC record available at https://lccn.loc.gov/2022010908
LC ebook record available at https://lccn.loc.gov/2022010909

DOI: 10.1093/med/9780197615768.001.0001

This material is not intended to be, and should not be considered, a substitute for medical or other
professional advice. Treatment for the conditions described in this material is highly dependent on the
individual circumstances. And, while this material is designed to offer accurate information with respect
to the subject matter covered and to be current as of the time it was written, research and knowledge about
medical and health issues is constantly evolving and dose schedules for medications are being revised
continually, with new side effects recognized and accounted for regularly. Readers must therefore always
check the product information and clinical procedures with the most up-to-date published product
information and data sheets provided by the manufacturers and the most recent codes of conduct and
safety regulation. The publisher and the authors make no representations or warranties to readers, express
or implied, as to the accuracy or completeness of this material. Without limiting the foregoing, the
publisher and the authors make no representations or warranties as to the accuracy or efficacy of the drug
dosages mentioned in the material. The authors and the publisher do not accept, and expressly disclaim,
any responsibility for any liability, loss, or risk that may be claimed or incurred as a consequence of the use
and/or application of any of the contents of this material.

1 3 5 7 9 8 6 4 2

Printed by Marquis, Canada

CONTENTS

FOREWORD

The recognition of posttraumatic stress disorder (PTSD) in the third edition of the American Psychiatric Association's *Diagnostic and Statistical Manual of Mental Disorders* (*DSM-III*) launched "traumatology"—a field comprising mental health professionals who study and treat survivors of traumatic stress. During the development of the *DSM-III*, Vietnam veterans and antiwar psychiatrists lobbied for the inclusion of Post-Vietnam Syndrome, noting that no extant diagnosis captured the delayed emergence of chronic signs and symptoms caused by the war. Although the *DSM-III* committee rejected a syndrome tied to a historical event, it approved the new diagnosis of PTSD after clinicians treating victims of rape, natural disasters, and the Holocaust emphasized that their patients experienced the same symptoms as those suffered by troubled Vietnam veterans. The ratification of PTSD in 1980 triggered an immense amount of research that continues to this day. Indeed, a recent bibliometric study indicated that the rate of publications on PTSD has greatly accelerated in the 21st century whereas the publication rates of other syndromes (e.g., panic disorder, social anxiety disorder) have remained stable.

PTSD mobilizes moral passions far more than other syndromes do. If someone develops bipolar disorder, there is no one at fault. But when a trauma victim develops PTSD, there is usually a perpetrator to blame. This can render otherwise ordinary scientific controversies especially explosive. For example, people skeptical of claims about hypnotically recovered "memories" of repressed memories of childhood sexual abuse have sometimes been accused of silencing the voices of survivors or having allied themselves with the perpetrators of sexual trauma. Traumatology has had no shortage of such controversies.

Joel Paris's latest book, *Myths of Trauma*, is a splendid introduction to these controversies. As a practicing psychiatrist specializing in the treatment of borderline personality disorder as well as a distinguished contributor to the scientific literature on personality psychopathology, he is ideally poised to dispel common misunderstandings—"myths"—about trauma and its consequences. Paris confirms that trauma is a common antecedent of other syndromes in addition to PTSD. He shows how its pathogenic impact is forever subject to the moderating influences of personality, temperament, and social context. The dramatic salience of serious stressors can sometimes eclipse other variables that amplify or attenuate the likelihood of survivors developing psychopathology or remaining resilient. Although many people experience acute symptoms in the immediate wake of trauma, most recover. PTSD is chiefly a failure of recovery.

Paris dispels confusions concerning dissociative identity disorder (multiple personality disorder), borderline personality, repressed (or dissociated) memories of trauma, premature enthusiasm for novel treatments for trauma survivors that lack empirical support, and the broadening of the concept of trauma far beyond its original boundaries. In addition to drawing on research from psychiatry and clinical psychology, he discusses key findings in epidemiology, history, genetics, cognitive psychology, and neuroscience.

In summary, Paris is a superb writer with an uncanny skill of writing about complex topics concisely and clearly. *Myths of Trauma* is the ideal source, especially for busy clinicians, for getting clear about the vicissitudes of trauma and its consequences.

Richard J. McNally, Ph.D.
Harvard University
Cambridge, Massachusetts
July 2022

INTRODUCTION

WHAT THIS BOOK IS ABOUT

Trauma is a term that describes damage to the mind caused by a distressing life event. Traumatic events, in and of themselves, are most certainly *not* a myth. Some events, such as shootings or rapes, are particularly likely to provoke posttraumatic symptoms. We need not lose sight of the fact that highly adverse life events can trigger serious psychopathology.

Even so, human life is full of adversity. This book will focus on the question of why some people fall ill while others show resilience in the face of adversity. The reason for the title of this book is that a mythology of trauma has been sometimes seen as implying that pathological responses are predictable from exposure alone. The large body of research reviewed in this book will show that they are not.

Moreover, most people will be exposed to traumatic events of some kind at several points in their lives. Some will go on to suffer from posttraumatic stress disorder (PTSD), a serious and potentially disabling mental disorder. This is one of the few categories of mental illness in which etiology is a criterion for making a diagnosis. Yet only about one in 10 of those exposed to most forms of trauma develop PTSD. This observation has been consistently confirmed in the scientific literature (Bromet et al., 2018). Research shows that trauma, while it is a trigger for PTSD symptoms, does not, by itself, cause the disorder. Thus, triggering events are a necessary but not a sufficient condition for this form of psychopathology. This book will attempt to explain why, and to draw some implications for clinical practice.

The idea that PTSD is almost entirely the result of exposure to adverse life events is problematic in another way. It leads to well-meaning treatment methods that are sympathetic to those who suffer adversity but seriously oversimplify the complex pathways to symptoms. This is particularly the case for childhood trauma. The evidence shows that trauma is a *nonspecific* risk factor for a large range of psychopathology, in which traumatic histories are usually associated with more severe outcomes. Yet trauma, by itself, is not a strong predictor of the large family of disorders that are associated with adverse life events.

Thus, while traumatic life events are well-established risks for many mental disorders, they do not, *by themselves*, cause PTSD. Instead, like most mental disorders, PTSD is the result of interactions between biological, psychological, and social risk factors. Thus, like most other mental disorders, PTSD has biopsychosocial origins. The complexity of these interactive pathways helps to explain why most people are resilient to life adversities of all kinds.

The key finding comes from research around the globe: *Most* people experience significant traumatic events in the course of a lifetime. The lifetime prevalence of these adversities is at least

75% (Breslau et al., 1998). Precise figures depend on what kind of experiences can be considered as being traumatic. And given the vagaries of human memory, the frequency of exposure is likely to be even higher. Those who have never known trauma are a lucky few. Yet the majority, who have been exposed but have not suffered serious consequences, can put adversity behind them and move on with their lives.

The point here is the large discrepancy between the frequency of exposure and the prevalence of PTSD. Ninety percent of people exposed to trauma will *not* develop the disorder (Sareen, 2014), which, once again, means that the proportion of those exposed who go on to develop PTSD is generally about 10%. The frequency can go as high as 20% in high-risk populations (Bromet et al., 2018), but that still leaves a large majority who never develop PTSD. It follows that *other* risk factors, and not trauma *alone*, need to be considered to explain how life events lead to symptoms. It also follows that treatment methods that focus exclusively on the processing of traumatic experiences fail to take these important coexisting risk factors into account, and such interventions may therefore be less effective.

Given the huge clinical and public profile of PTSD, it is important to acknowledge that while trauma is a scientific issue, it is also a highly emotional one. Most of us strongly sympathize with victims. That is why I need to clarify that I am *not* arguing that traumatic events are unimportant, or that they have no effect on the risk for symptoms. Of course they do. What I *am* saying is that in order to understand trauma, we need to think about cause and effect in a complex and multivariate context. Thus, trauma is a nonspecific factor that interacts with many other risks and can be best understood within a biopsychosocial model. We need to consider PTSD, like other mental disorders, as the outcome of interactions among biological, psychosocial, and social risk factors.

WHY I HAVE WRITTEN THIS BOOK

I am not a researcher on PTSD. My career has focused on personality disorders, particularly borderline personality disorder (BPD). But there are major theories about BPD that focus on the role of childhood trauma, and some have thought of the disorder as a variant of PTSD. My clinical experience in this domain, and my reading of the scientific literature, have led me reject that conclusion, and to adopt multivariate models of BPD that focus on gene–environment interactions (Paris, 2020a, 2020d).

Research on the causes of BPD has long been affected by simplistic theories that attribute complex problems in mood regulation, identity, impulsivity, and interpersonal relationships to childhood trauma, without considering a broader range of biological, psychosocial, or social factors. This trend toward a "trauma focus" in therapy and a redefinition of BPD as "complex PTSD" are problematic and can have a negative effect on practice. These troubling developments have led me to review a broader literature on the effects of traumatic events and on what else (besides exposure) causes PTSD.

I have also written this book because of my concern that clinicians treating patients with PTSD or related symptoms fail to take into account the complexity of posttraumatic outcomes. If adverse events can be found in a patient's history, therapists may be tempted to attribute problems of all kinds to the effects of exposure. This rush to judgment vastly oversimplifies the complex pathways to disorder, and it constitutes one of the main myths of trauma.

Since the word "myth" is in the title of this book, let me explain what I mean by it. Over 20 years ago, I wrote a book entitled *Myths of Childhood* (Paris, 2000a). In that volume, I used this word to describe ideas about putative causes of mental disorders originating in childhood that are commonly held by clinicians (and by the general public) but that are not supported by scientific evidence. One of these myths is that traumatic events, particularly when they occur early in life, affect everyone in much the same way and are a major cause and predictor of adult psychopathology. This book will show that the pathological outcomes are not solely predicted by exposure to trauma but are affected by traits *internal* to individuals that are associated with a vulnerability to mental disorders.

These issues have profound implications for clinical work. Because I treat people with BPD, I actively practice psychotherapy and have spent many decades treating patients with histories of childhood trauma. I always work with patients to make sense of these experiences. But my research on the causes of BPD, including studies of the role of child abuse and family dysfunction, has led me to approach this problem from a different perspective, leading me to draw different conclusions.

For example, our research group (Laporte et al., 2012) recruited 56 women with BPD along with their sisters. Although these siblings grew up in the same family, and described many of the same adverse experiences, only three pairs were concordant for BPD, while 53 were not. The key point was that the sisters differed greatly in personality trait profiles, supporting the view that vulnerability to trauma, based on both genetic and nontraumatic environmental factors, plays a major role in the risk for BPD.

As important as it is, childhood adversity need not be the main or only subject of discussion in the psychotherapy of BPD. Nor should a personality disorder, which has broad effects on emotion regulation and impulsivity, be reclassified as a form of PTSD. Instead, the impact of life events needs to be understood in the context of two larger issues. The first is that trauma has a stronger pathogenic effect on those whose personality traits make them more vulnerable. The other is that traumatic events in childhood are associated with broader problems of family dysfunction and emotional neglect that are themselves a major source of vulnerability, denying children the support they need to rise above adversity.

This book will recommend a similar approach to understanding PTSD in adults. Again, what needs to be explained is why only a minority of those exposed to highly adverse events develop posttraumatic symptoms. I will review evidence showing that the impact of traumatic events on individuals is greatly amplified by temperamental vulnerability, by a past history of trauma, and by weak social supports.

In summary, while trauma is an important risk factor for many forms of psychopathology, it is not, by itself, consistently predictive of *any* mental disorder. Adverse life events must be acknowledged and explored but need not be the main focus of psychological treatment. This book will suggest a different way of addressing these problems, one that takes personality and life course into account.

THE ROOTS OF RESILIENCE

The capacity to not develop mental disorders after trauma is called *resilience* (i.e., the ability to rise above adversity). Nietzsche no doubt exaggerated when he argued that what does not kill us makes us stronger. Yet positive outcomes, or what Rutter et al. (2012) call "steeling," do occur. This increase in resilience after trauma has also been called *posttraumatic growth* (Tedeschi et al., 2018). Yet most outcomes fall within a range between a lasting and strong reaction and a temporary and weak one. Those who are most vulnerable to adversity become the patients clinicians see in therapy. They do not see the majority of people who have experienced traumatic events, because they do not suffer enough to present to clinics, and because many find a way to go on with their lives.

While it is important to assess the impact of traumatic events in light of their severity, we can frame them within a larger biopsychosocial context. This allows us to consider the crucial role of resilience in protecting people from psychopathology. This book will place emphasis on genetic variations and predispositions that influence how people process life events (Plomin, 2018). In that light, I will also explore the concept of *differential susceptibility to the environment* (Belsky & Pluess, 2009). As we will see, this is a similar construct to the personality trait of Neuroticism (Costa & Widiger, 2015). People who are more susceptible to their environment are much more likely to develop mental disorders, including PTSD (Bowman & Yehuda, 2004).

Put simply, differential susceptibility means that some people are thin-skinned, while others are thick-skinned (with most falling somewhere in between). Those who are less susceptible tend to have transitory symptoms or none at all. While those who are thin-skinned tend to be more severely affected by adversity, this group, because of their higher sensitivity, are also more likely to benefit from a *positive* environment. That finding places differential susceptibility in an evolutionary context, and helps explain why these traits remain in the gene pool.

Let us consider some examples. Research consistently shows that trauma does not necessarily come out of the blue. For example, children who are sexually or physically abused have often received insufficient love from their families; emotional neglect makes them more likely to be exposed to and susceptible to traumatic events (Johnson et al., 2000). Since coexisting psychological risk factors influence response to adversity, we should view the overall risk of disorder in those who have been traumatized as reflecting interactive pathways (Kraemer et al., 2001).

We see similar predisposing factors for adults who develop PTSD after a traumatic event. Again, genetic vulnerability and personality profiles, as well as histories of multiple stressors with cumulative effects, help explain why only one out of 10 people exposed to trauma ever develop PTSD. Thus, even when trauma is implicated in the etiology of a mental disorder, it rarely accounts for a larger proportion of the variance in outcome (Horwitz, 2018; McNally, 2003).

All these research findings teach us to avoid thinking about trauma in isolation. They also show why we should avoid seeing trauma as one thing rather than many different things. These details can be described as the *parameters* of trauma. In childhood trauma, the main parameters include the nature of the event, the length of exposure, and the identity of perpetrators (Browne & Finkelhor, 1986). In adult trauma, the most important parameters concern whether adverse events involve interpersonal violence, rape, or threats to life (Sareen, 2014). The more severe these parameters, the more likely it is that PTSD will be an outcome.

IMPLICATIONS FOR CLINICAL PRACTICE

This book aims to warn clinicians about the tendency to overdiagnose PTSD, or to explain too much about patients from traumatic events in their life history (Paris, 2020d). This error becomes more likely when clinicians see trauma as an all-powerful force that has the capacity to override resilience. It can also lead to therapeutic interventions that explore the past rather than focus on present difficulties, distracting clinicians and patients from the primary tasks of therapy.

What accounts for the tendency to give too much weight to traumatic events? The first problem is that clinicians and researchers who observe and measure adverse experiences usually do so in clinical populations. Drawing broad conclusions from patients in treatment biases observations in favor of negative consequences and oversimplifies the role of risk factors. To avoid this error, we should not rely entirely on clinical samples but rather should obtain data on trauma in community populations.

The second problem is that research often measures life events with questionnaires or interviews that are cross-sectional and that depend on accurate recall of past events. That is why we need more longitudinal studies of people exposed to trauma. As this book will show, existing studies of this kind show that memories of these events can change over time, and that outcomes are not highly predictable.

The third problem is that even when research is conducted in the community, it often fails to measure the psychosocial context of life events or the coexisting risk factors with which they are associated. The result is that researchers end up taking insufficient account of differences in susceptibility to the environment.

The fourth problem derives from political and social forces that influence our view of PTSD, creating a "culture of trauma" (Horwitz, 2018). In the heyday of psychoanalysis, many clinicians took it for granted that childhood trauma is a powerful risk factor for adult psychopathology. These ideas remain influential and have spread to other academic disciplines (such as history and biography). While current theories of child development tend to focus more on genetic risk, they are still incomplete, failing to examine the interactions between genes and environment that best predict the development of psychological symptoms (Rutter, 2006). Finally, political movements that aim to promote social justice may be influenced by a wish to validate adverse life experiences.

Myths of trauma can be partly understood as a reflection of an era in which virtuous thinking focuses on the suffering of all who have been badly treated and/or marginalized. This is not, of course, to say that mistreatment and marginalization are not painful—they usually are. And adverse life events *do* need to be explored in therapy. The question is whether it makes scientific sense to think of trauma as independent of other risk factors, or outside a larger context of adverse events that have, over the long term, cumulative effects. In this context, therapy need not be "trauma-focused" but should concern itself with life histories as a whole. In this way, treatment needs to give priority to the present and future, not just to the past.

Unfortunately, the effects of trauma are surrounded by myths that carry a strong emotional impact and that insert a measure of *drama* into the routine work of psychotherapy. Thus, a *narrative* tends to develop around trauma (Young, 1995). The result can be a failure to benefit patients who seek help for current problems; instead, they are provided with well-meaning but misguided therapy. I will suggest alternatives using psychotherapies that are based on better empirical evidence.

In summary, the main themes of the book can be summarized as follows:

1. Trauma has become a catchword for many kinds of adverse experiences; this is a construct that needs to be more narrowly and precisely defined.

2. Traumatic events have always been a part of human life, and most people are notably resilient to adversity.

3. Exposure to trauma is only one risk factor for PTSD, and not always the most important one. The disorder can only be understood in a biopsychosocial model, taking into account genetic vulnerability, personality trait profiles, previous adversities, and levels of social support.

4. Trauma has become a political issue that interferes with unbiased scientific study of its effects.

5. The concept of repressed and recovered memories of traumatic events is scientifically invalid.

6. The wide comorbidity of PTSD, particularly when symptoms are chronic, means that it cannot be considered as a specific category with a specific treatment, and that treatment for patients should be broadly biopsychosocial.

7. Complex PTSD is a new but problematic diagnosis, and most of its features can be better explained by personality disorders.

8. Several evidence-based methods of treatment for PTSD have been developed, but their effectiveness is no greater than that of standard cognitive-behavioral therapy.

9. Understanding experiences of trauma has a place in the treatment of PTSD, but excessive focus on processing memories can be a mistake.

10. A focus on trauma narratives can also work against the interests of patients by encouraging victimhood instead of a sense of competence and agency.

Thus, based on a large research literature, I will offer a view of how contemporary theory and practice in mental health need to be broadened to determine the true effects of traumatic events in adult life. This book will offer a more complex and multidimensional view of PTSD than is currently held by clinicians, patients, or the educated public.

ACKNOWLEDGMENTS

Lise Laporte read an earlier version of this book and provided detailed and insightful feedback. Allan Young read several chapters of a draft and also offered helpful comments.

Chapter 1

Does Trauma Cause Posttraumatic Stress Disorder?

PROBLEMS IN DEFINING CRITERIA FOR POSTTRAUMATIC STRESS DISORDER

Posttraumatic stress disorder (PTSD) was introduced into the standard diagnostic classification over 40 years ago, in the third edition of the *Diagnostic and Statistical Manual of Mental Disorders* (DSM-III; American Psychiatric Association, 1980). While there were some precedents for this construct, historical forces, particularly the Vietnam War and its aftermath, were a major factor in its adoption.

PTSD, unlike most categories in the DSM system, is linked to a specific etiology. Exposure to traumatic stress is, by definition, a necessary condition for PTSD. But the manual fails to emphasize that exposure is not sufficient. Research repeatedly shows that only a subgroup of individuals exposed to the same adverse events will develop posttraumatic symptoms (Bryant, 2019).

In DSM-5 (American Psychiatric Association, 2013), PTSD can be diagnosed if all of the following criteria are met:

Criterion A: Definition of the stressor (exposure to death, threatened death, actual or threatened injury or sexual violence; through direct exposure, witnessing or learning of a trauma, or indirect exposure in course of professional duties)

Criterion B: Intrusion symptoms (at least one: upsetting memories, nightmares, flashbacks, distress or physical reactivity after exposure to reminders)

Criterion C: Avoidance symptoms (at least one: trauma-related thoughts or feelings, or external reminders)

Criterion D: Negative alterations in cognition and mood (at least two: problems with memory, negative thoughts, self-blame, negative mood, decreased interest in activities, isolation, loss of positive affect)

Criterion E: Alterations in arousal and reactivity (irritability, risky behavior, hypervigilance, startle reactions difficulty concentrating, difficulty sleeping)

Criterion F: Duration (at least 1 month)

Criterion G: Functional significance (distress or impairment)

Criterion H: Exclusion (not due to another disorder)

DSM-5 also lists two possible specifiers for subgroups: (1) the presence of notable dissociative symptoms and (2) a delay in the onset of full symptoms.

This definition of PTSD has a long history behind it, and in some ways the construct has become broader over time. The most crucial issue has been a gradual expansion of Criterion A. DSM-5 made an attempt to narrow it somewhat, but the problem remains.

PTSD AND CONCEPT CREEP

In DSM-III (American Psychiatric Association, 1980) the definition of a stressor was an event that "would evoke significant symptoms of distress in almost everyone" and that was "generally outside the range of usual human experience." In the revised version (DSM-III-R; American Psychiatric Association, 1987), the definition required exposure to death, threatened death, or actual or threatened serious injury or violence. In DSM-IV (American Psychiatric Association, 1994), this criterion was broadened to include indirect exposure, such as witnessing a trauma, learning that a relative or close friend was exposed to a trauma, or working in a field where trauma is common.

The definition of a stressor in DSM-5 (American Psychiatric Association, 2013) remains overly broad. As defined in Criterion A, it requires "exposure to actual or threatened death, serious injury, or sexual violence in one (or more) of the following ways: directly experiencing the traumatic event, witnessing, in person, the event as it occurred to others, learning that a violent or accidental event occurred to a close family member or close friend, or repeated exposure to aversive details of the traumatic event (e.g., first responders collecting remains, or police officers investigating child abuse)." The main narrowing of the criterion was that exposure due to watching a traumatic event on television no longer meets criteria for a stressor.

Thus, the definition of a stressor in DSM's Criterion A has changed in consecutive editions of the manual: It started with life-threatening events and gradually broadened out to include all sorts of adverse events, sometimes even including just hearing about one. This expansion of what kinds of events can be called "traumatic" is a good example of *concept creep* (Haslam, 2016; McNally, 2016). In other words, one starts with a narrow definition that gradually broadens. Concept creep is one of the main reasons for overdiagnosis of all kinds of disorders in psychiatry (Paris, 2020c).

The definition of PTSD on the International Classification of Diseases (ICD-11; World Health Organization, 2019) is more succinct and relatively more conservative:

> Post-traumatic stress disorder (PTSD) is a disorder that may develop following exposure to an extremely threatening or horrific event or series of events. It is characterized by all of the following: 1) re-experiencing the traumatic event or events in the present in the form of vivid intrusive memories, flashbacks, or nightmares. These are typically accompanied by strong or overwhelming emotions, particularly fear or horror, and strong physical sensations; 2) avoidance of thoughts and memories of the event or events, or avoidance of activities, situations, or people reminiscent of the event or events; and 3) persistent perceptions of heightened current threat, for example as indicated by hypervigilance or an enhanced startle reaction to stimuli such as unexpected noises. The symptoms persist for at least several weeks and cause significant impairment in personal, family, social, educational, occupational or other important areas of functioning.

Central to this definition is the principle that a core component of PTSD is a reexperiencing of the memories of the traumatic event in the present. However, unlike DSM-5, ICD-11 avoids focusing on symptoms that are not specific to PTSD, and that could equally well lead to a mood or an anxiety disorder. This change reflects the aim of making PTSD more specific (Brewin et al., 2017) and reducing the frequency of the diagnosis (Cloitre et al., 2014).

Up to now, given that so much of the research on PTSD has come from North America, the DSM definitions have predominated. Thus, as different cutoff points have been used to determine "caseness," concept creep has led to an overall broadening of what can be considered "traumatic" (North et al., 2009). In some community studies (e.g., Breslau et al., 1991), even events as common as divorce or job loss were considered to be triggers for PTSD. There is much less controversy about whether war, rape, violence, and other severe traumas should be viewed as stressors.

These diagnostic problems have made the precise prevalence of PTSD difficult to measure. Nonetheless, large-scale epidemiological studies have been conducted in the community to determine the prevalence of mental disorders commonly seen in clinical settings. Reports based on the Epidemiological Catchment Area survey in the 1980s for DSM-III–defined PTSD (Robins & Regier, 1991) yielded a lifetime prevalence of 1% for PTSD. However, using DSM-IV criteria, the National Comorbidity Survey (Kessler et al., 1995) reported a lifetime prevalence of 7.6%—a vast increase. The National Comorbidity Survey Replication in the early 2000s (Kessler et al., 2005a, 2005b), also based on DSM-IV, found a similar rate: 6.8% (with 10.4% in women, but only 5% in men). Other large-scale surveys have reported rates of 8% to 9% (Breslau et al., 1991, 1998; Kilpatrick et al., 2013). These rates remain notably high but are lower than high lifetime rates of exposure to trauma. This trend can lead to an overdiagnosis of the disorder and an overuse of trauma-focused therapies.

DIAGNOSES ON THE BORDERS OF PTSD

Acute Stress Disorder

In addition to PTSD, the DSM-5 includes a diagnosis of acute stress disorder, which describes reactions occurring immediately after trauma exposure that last for less than a month. This diagnosis was introduced in DSM-IV as a means to describe distressed people who could not be diagnosed in the initial phases but who might still be at risk for full PTSD. However, subsequent longitudinal studies indicated that the diagnosis is only a modest predictor of that outcome; in one sample, at least half of those who eventually developed PTSD had never initially met the criteria for acute stress disorder (Bryant & Harvey, 1998). Also, people who develop PTSD do not necessarily display the same features in the acute phase as they do later on. In DSM-5, the diagnosis of acute stress disorder does not require any specific symptom or symptom clusters to be present but states that nine of 14 features should be present.

Complex PTSD

ICD-11 (World Health Organization 2019) has introduced a new diagnostic construct: *complex PTSD*. To receive this diagnosis, one needs to present core PTSD symptoms, and in addition, disturbances in self-identity (a negative self-concept), emotional dysregulation (emotional reactivity, violent outbursts), and persistent difficulties in relationships. This syndrome overlaps greatly with persons with borderline personality disorder who also have an abuse history. Using the word "complex" is an attempt to acknowledge that repeated trauma is more important that single incidents. But the danger is that trauma will be considered the only cause of what we have up to now been calling a personality disorder. I will discuss these issues in more detail in Chapter 7.

TRAUMATIC AND NONTRAUMATIC RISKS FOR PTSD

The drama of traumatic life events has distracted clinicians from considering the broader context in which PTSD develops. The discrepancy between exposure to stressors and the development of the disorder requires attention to other, nontraumatic risk factors.

Again, the etiology of PTSD can be best understood in the same way as other categories of mental disorder: that is, by using a *biopsychosocial model* (Engel, 1980). This term is used to describe interactions among genetic diatheses, life events, and social stressors that can lead to psychopathology (Paris, 2020d). Since research shows that trauma is a necessary but not sufficient condition for the development of PTSD, taking these interactions into account is crucial.

What predisposes a minority of those exposed to trauma to develop the disorder? Part of the explanation is that crucial risk factors can be present *prior* to exposure to adverse life events. Many of the risks are the same as have been documented in other mental disorders. They include female gender, a lower socioeconomic level, a prior mental disorder, a family history of mental disorders, and past trauma (Horwitz, 2018). Horwitz also noted that the subjective response to trauma plays a major role. Thus, catastrophic appraisals about the outcome of an event are associated with later severity. For this reason, both the pretraumatic and posttraumatic environments are important, with low social support and ongoing stressors contributing to overall risk. However, none of these factors by themselves, or any combination of them, can definitively predict who will develop PTSD and who will not. Most likely, all play a role, and multiple risks lead most consistently to a cumulative effect.

Severity of trauma is an important parameter affecting relationships between exposure and outcome. This has been shown in community populations of civilians experiencing traumatic events (Breslau et al., 1991) and in veterans with a history of combat exposure (Schlenger et al., 1992), as well as in populations who have experienced rape (Chivers-Wilson, 2006). Severity is related to earlier definitions of Criterion A—that is, events that are violent and/or life-threatening.

Community research shows that when traumatic events are life-threatening or involve violence, the prevalence of the disorder goes up, with nearly 25% of exposed individuals likely to develop PTSD. In contrast, rates are lower when less severe events are involved. For example, in the urban sample studied by Breslau et al. (1991), which included a very wide range of adverse experiences, the likelihood of risk for PTSD after exposure for all events was 9%. Thus even for higher-risk stressors, data consistently show that at least three quarters of those exposed to such events will not develop the clinical disorder (Horwitz, 2018).

Again, we need to keep in mind that traumatic experiences are ubiquitous. Breslau et al. (1991) found that 40% of a population in Detroit were exposed to at least one life event that involved a serious threat per year, and that 90% experienced such events over a lifetime. Data from the National Comorbidity Survey (Kessler et al., 1995) showed that while exposure to a specific trauma plays a role, it is not as important a predictor as prior trauma and the cumulative effects of multiple life stressors. This relationship was later quantified in a large-scale study in which the path-analytic correlation between severity of exposure and outcome was only 0.2 (Seedat & Stein, 2001).

The Environmental Risk Twin Study (E-Risk) studied a cohort of twins in the United Kingdom followed longitudinally from childhood to adulthood (Lewis et al., 2019). The results showed a similar cross-sectional prevalence of exposure to trauma as in other studies: 31%. The prevalence of PTSD was much lower than that (7.8%), and, as in other studies, was associated with exposures that involved interpersonal threats or violence. Once again, these are the features of a traumatic event that are most likely to trigger PTSD.

Many other studies have confirmed that interpersonal violence leads to higher rates of PTSD. For example, the World Mental Health Surveys (Kessler et al., 2017) found that physical or sexual violence raises risk, and that rates were markedly lower in PTSD following natural disasters (typically 5% to 10%) than after sexual assault (13% to 15%). In the same survey, rates of PTSD associated with intimate partner violence were notably higher than those associated with war and terrorism. These findings suggests that the interpersonal context of an event can be as important for our social brains as whether or not it threatens life.

Another line of evidence pointing to a lack of specificity between trauma and PTSD is that traumatic events are a risk factor for many diagnoses, including depression, anxiety, and personality disorders (Horwitz, 2018). Moreover, PTSD has a high comorbidity with depression, anxiety, and substance use and shares genetic risks with these disorders (Sareen, 2014). This finding points to a lack of specificity between stressors and pathological outcomes. It suggests that the disorder that develops after trauma depends as much on individual predisposition as on stressors alone.

All these findings point to interactions and complexity in the causal pathways to PTSD. It is fair to conclude that the nature of adverse life events is only one of many factors that account for discrepancies between exposure and outcome. Trauma is a risk factor for PTSD but does not act alone.

STRESSORS THAT CARRY A HIGH RISK

Let us now examine research on the effects of stressors that carry a particularly high risk. Note again the finding of Breslau et al. (1998) that while the conditional risk of PTSD after traumatic events of any kind was 9.2%, the rate after assaultive violence was more than twice as high (20.9%). Rape is the best example. Estimates of risk for PTSD following rape differ depending on samples (Sareen, 2014) but tend to cluster around 25%, one of the highest rates reported for any life event. Nonetheless, since the majority of those exposed to rape do not develop posttraumatic symptoms, individual differences in vulnerability must also be important predictors of outcome (Bowman & Yehuda, 2004).

Long-term follow-up studies are needed to determine whether stressors that lead to higher rates of acute PTSD are also associated with greater chronicity. Surprisingly, only a few long-term studies of rape victims have been carried out, and most have been limited by follow-up times of a year or less. The longest, with a mean follow-up time of 4.6 years (Regehr & Marziali, 1999), reported that 21% retained at least one PTSD symptom, but most no longer met criteria for the disorder. These authors also found that chronicity of symptoms after rape was associated with prior deficits in interpersonal functioning.

For an even higher potential risk, consider studies of Holocaust survivors. By and large, research has documented higher rates of posttraumatic symptoms, but these features are only found in a minority of cases, are not universal, and do not necessarily meet criteria for PTSD (Yehuda & Lehmer, 2018). As confirmed by a large-scale meta-analysis (Barel et al., 2010), Holocaust survivors had more symptoms, even though their overall level of functioning was close to normal. Similar findings emerged from a study of survivors in the community who had not sought clinical treatment (Eaton et al., 1982). Essentially, Holocaust survivors bear psychological scars but do not necessarily develop the full clinical picture of PTSD.

The next example concerns a population that has been of particular interest to clinicians and investigators: Vietnam veterans, whose mental health stimulated a very large body of research (McNally, 2007). Studies in community populations soon after the war did not find a high rate of PTSD after combat exposure, yet follow-up studies of clinical populations attending Veterans Administration clinics have found PTSD to be more prevalent and more chronic (Horwitz, 2018). This discrepancy has led to some controversy.

The National Vietnam Veterans Readjustment Study was a large-scale study of this population. The lifetime prevalence of PTSD in this cohort was estimated to be 31% among male theater veterans and 26% among females, augmented by a prevalence of partial PTSD of 11.1% in males and 7.8% in females (Kulka et al., 1990; Weiss et al., 1992). These data suggest that nearly a third of those who had served in the war were still experiencing clinically significant distress and disability years later.

Yet even longer after the end of the war, the cohort was revisited in the National Vietnam Veterans Longitudinal Study (Marmar et al., 2015). By this time, the prevalence of PTSD had fallen sharply and was only 1.2% in males and 3.9% in females, although 36.7% met criteria for major depression. (We cannot say for sure whether depression was war-related or whether there was a selection bias in who went to Vietnam and who did not.)

Another confusing finding was that only about half of Vietnam veterans claiming benefits due to trauma *ever* saw combat, even if they were assigned to a war zone (Dohrenwend et al., 2019).

Dorhenwend et al. (2006) reexamined data in 260 veterans, cross-checked military records, and found that combat exposure could not always be validated. This was particularly the case for women, most of whom were nurses. Given that access to health care was a benefit for those who presented to a public health care system, it is possible that some veterans were at risk for the symptoms PTSD for reasons not related to military service (Horwitz, 2018).

Even among those who did have significant combat exposure, predispositions can be important. Heritability of symptoms associated with PTSD can be measured in behavioral genetic research, in which comparisons are made between monozygotic and dizygotic twins. A study of twins serving in Vietnam found that after controlling for combat exposure, *each* symptom in DSM-III–defined PTSD was separately heritable, with about 30% of the variance related to genetic differences (True et al., 1993). Moreover, exposure to trauma can itself have a genetic component related to traits that promote risk-taking (Lykken, 1995).

There are also cross-national differences in the prevalence of PTSD associated with combat exposure. The prevalence of the disorder is relatively lower, for example, in Israel (Shalev et al., 2000). That could be because military service is more honored in countries that depend on soldiers for their survival, as opposed to volunteers or draftees serving in unpopular foreign wars. In the Iraq war, the prevalence of PTSD was much lower among UK soldiers than Americans (Jones & Wessely, 2005), but the nature of combat was a factor, given that British soldiers had much less exposure to danger. American soldiers in the Iraq war developed the disorder at rates ranging from 10% to 17% (Greenberg et al., 2011), and this rate could have been related either to the nature of combat (guerilla warfare) or to preexisting differences related to the recruitment of a volunteer army.

Monetary compensation for combat exposure may also play a role in PTSD. The number seeking government compensation was much higher for veterans of the Iraq and Afghanistan wars than it was in the Vietnam era (McNally & Frueh, 2013). All of these wars were unpopular, but compensation can sometimes become an entitlement.

Since severity of trauma is a predictor of PTSD, much research has focused on those who are particularly likely to face threats to life due to the nature of their work. One such group are firefighters. But while firefighters do have higher rates of PTSD, the picture changes if you evaluate them *before* they are exposed to trauma. Yehuda and McFarlane (1995) found that the rate of PTSD in Australian bushfire fighters was high but, when followed over time, was strongly related to baseline levels of trait neuroticism, and to previous histories of psychological symptoms.

Another high-risk occupation is being a police officer. In one study of this group, the rate of PTSD was 13%, strongly related to exposure to life-threatening situations (Robinson et al., 1997). Similar findings in those involved in law enforcement have been reported by other research groups (Maguen et al., 2009). It is again notable that most of those in high-risk occupations who were exposed did not develop PTSD. Some were highly vulnerable, while others were not. It follows that PTSD is a more complex disorder than we usually think.

Even after the most severe events, the pattern is similar. Among those who were in danger during 9/11, the prevalence of PTSD was 7.4% (Lowell et al., 2018). Similar effects have observed after the recent COVID-19 pandemic (Yuan et al., 2021). These levels are in line with the more general findings about the prevalence of PTSD after exposure.

Finally, it is important to note that women in the general population have almost twice the prevalence of PTSD as do men. The most likely explanation derives from gender differences in person-ality traits: Women have much higher scores on neuroticism and react more strongly to stressful events (Weisberg et al., 2011).

PTSD AROUND THE WORLD

PTSD is not just a North American or European problem: The World Mental Health Surveys (Kessler et al., 2017) reported life-time prevalence rates around the globe of 13.0% to 20.4% for women and 6.2% to 8.2% for men. These surveys have observed higher 12-month prevalence rates in high-income countries (e.g., Northern Ireland, 3.8%; United States, 2.5%; New Zealand, 2.1%) than in low- and middle-income countries (e.g., Colombia, 0.3%; Mexico, 0.3%). This finding might reflect the fact that while the lives of people in poorer countries may be experienced as "normally" traumatic, those living in developed countries are more likely to see trauma as unusual.

There is evidence that the prevalence of PTSD is higher in cer-tain ethnic groups, such as Hispanics and African Americans in the United States (Kessler et al., 2005a). These findings may be due to differential access to health resources, ethnic discrimination, or other socioeconomic factors. Occupations that involve exposure to trauma (the military, police, and firefighters) are more likely to put workers at risk for PTSD (Lee et al., 2020). Finally, commu-nity studies find that women are generally more at risk than men, with the important exception of war veterans and police (Tolin & Foa, 2006).

PTSD overlaps with other mental disorders and does not nec-essarily present as a single diagnosis. This overlap is usually called "comorbidity," which describes the presence of multiple disorders in the same patient. However, what multiple diagnoses actually reflect is the lack of precision and specificity of DSM-based diagnostic criteria (Paris, 2020a). If you follow the manual closely, almost all your patients will have more than one diagnosis. And PTSD overlaps with many other disorders: Epidemiological studies show that almost all patients with PTSD have comorbid diagnoses, particularly depression, anxiety disorders, and substance use disorders (Kessler et al., 2005a), as well as personality disorders (Paris, 2000a). Comorbidity is particularly high when PTSD is chronic and does not respond well to treatment (Brady et al., 2000).

Some of these comorbidities will have been present prior to trauma exposure. The risk factors for common mental disorders such as major depression or anxiety tend to be similar to those for PTSD, including both heritability (Stein et al., 2002) and personality profiles (Jang et al., 2003). Thus, people who are predisposed to react to traumatic events more intensely can have a wide range of symptoms. This suggests that trauma need not be the primary etiological factor when comorbidity is high. While exposure does increase the overall prevalence of psychological symptoms, only some patients will meet formal PTSD criteria. Given the range of disorders that can emerge after exposure to trauma, PTSD can sometimes be a "point of transition" to other diagnoses (Yehuda & McFarlane, 1995).

PTSD shows individual variation in its course and outcome. It does not necessarily follow a linear course but can fluctuate over time. Network analysis, which measures the strength of relationships between symptoms, shows that PTSD gradually develops over time before remitting (McNally, 2017). In the acute phase after trauma, symptoms are loosely interconnected, but they become more closely related with other characteristic features (reexperiencing, active avoidance) as time progresses. We do not know whether this is a naturalistic development or whether it reflects priming by therapists who closely follow the diagnostic criteria and regularly inquire about them.

All these findings from research suggest that PTSD is not necessarily a discrete diagnosis but rather lies within a broad spectrum of *internalizing disorders* that affect mood and personality (Costa & Widiger, 2015). Moreover, the inconsistent relationship between past traumas and present functioning points to the need for a broader model.

BUILDING A BROADER MODEL OF PTSD

While research yields a large body of evidence supporting relationships between trauma and psychopathology, we should not confuse correlation with causation. By and large, traumatic histories are best understood as *markers* for broader risks, derived from pathways that are complex, interactive, and biopsychosocial.

Few risk factors, whether biological or psychosocial, are specific to *any* mental disorder. These etiological complexities also apply to the most severe and clinically important categories of illness. Thus schizophrenia and bipolar disorders, separated over a century ago by Kraepelin, are associated with shared genetic and environmental risks (Lichtenstein et al., 2009). Much the same is true for common mental disorders such as anxiety and depression, categories that share an association with high Neuroticism (Goldberg & Goodyer, 2005).

As DSM manuals steadily broadened the definition of PTSD, this diagnosis tended to become more comorbid with related disorders. Ultimately these difficulties reflect the limitations of diagnostic validity in current practice. We do not know whether current classification systems will still be considered valid in another half-century or will be regarded as historical relics. Even so, the construct of PTSD remains useful because it describes a characteristic clinical picture, for which treatments have been devised that have some degree of specificity.

Keep in mind that exposure to traumatic events early in life or later in development also constitutes a nonspecific risk factor for many mental disorders and is far from specific to PTSD. The list includes schizophrenia (Bentall, 2003), depressive and/or anxiety disorders (Amstadter et al., 2012), bipolar disorders (Rowland & Marwaha, 2018), substance use disorders (Kendler & Prescott, 2007), and personality disorders (Paris, 2020a).

In summary, since PTSD is only one possible outcome of traumatic experiences, the way the diagnostic criteria for this condition are written, focusing almost entirely on the nature of the traumatic exposure and specific symptoms that follow exposure, is misleading. PTSD is determined as much by internal as by external factors. Personality traits, most particularly Neuroticism, accounts for a great deal of the vulnerability to PTSD. Neuroticism measures the intensity and course of reactions to stressful events (Costa & Widiger, 2015). It also has important physiological correlates related to autonomic activation (Pineles et al., 2017). Thus, the stronger your reaction to stress, the more likely you are to develop the disorder. The next chapter will explore the sources of individual variation that determine the risk for PTSD.

Chapter 2

Individual Differences in Response to Trauma

PERSONALITY TRAITS AND THE PSYCHOLOGICAL IMMUNE SYSTEM

Very few diseases in medicine affect every person exposed to the same risks in the same way. In 2020–2022, a pandemic raged around the world, but not everyone who was infected developed symptoms, and among those who did, illness severity varied greatly. If the course of infectious diseases depends on variations in the immune system that reflect genetic differences and past exposures, the same could well be true for mental disorders.

In this light, it is useful to define a *psychological immune system* that is strongly related to personality trait profiles (Millon & Davis, 1995). This concept describes innate and acquired variabilities in how strongly people respond to adverse life experiences. Due to natural selection, our minds are programmed to deal with environmental challenges, but the ability to do so varies greatly between individuals.

Let us return to the seminal article by Belsky and Pluess (2009) that introduced the construct of differential susceptibility to the environment. Individual differences lead to a wide range of responses to environmental challenges. At one end of the spectrum, some people will be affected by almost any kind of adversity, and they are easily overstimulated or upended by life events. At the other end of the spectrum are people who are able to compartmentalize or ignore such events, and who have a much higher threshold for emotional response.

Differential susceptibility parallels the well-known psychological construct of scores on the broad trait dimension of Neuroticism (Costa & Widiger, 2015). This trait measures sensitivity to the environment, which lies on a continuum, leaving plenty of room between two extremes. (Although Neuroticism is almost always measured through self-report, the same characteristics emerge from research based on observer ratings.)

We see these trait differences every day in clinical practice, and they help account for the fact that some find changes in their circumstances to be stressful, while others are less affected and/or more resilient to life events. The most useful way of assessing these differences in environmental susceptibility is to measure personality trait profiles (Paris, 2020d).

BEHAVIOR GENETICS AND THE CRUCIAL ROLE OF NEUROTICISM

As has become usual in psychopathology, theories about etiology need to begin with genetics. The principle is that some people are more vulnerable by temperament to developing symptoms after facing adversity, while others are less vulnerable (Belsky & Pluess, 2009).

Behavioral genetic research provides some of the strongest evidence for heritable risks for mental disorders. This method, based on differences in concordance for psychological outcomes in monozygotic versus dizygotic twins, shows that genetic predispositions influence almost every trait or mental disorder (Knopik et al., 2017). It should be noted that the precise level of heritability will not be found in all environments, but there will always be a significant component.

This line of research shows that almost all mental disorders are partially heritable, with genetic variations accounting for at least 40% of outcome variance (Plomin, 2018). The same level of heritability also applies to personality traits (Livesley et al., 1998). Similarly, genetic variations influence whether people who are exposed to trauma are likely to develop posttraumatic stress disorder (PTSD), irrespective of the nature of a stressor.

Yet while heritable influences can be risk factors for psychopathology, they are rarely, by themselves, a complete explanation for disorders. About half of the variance in personality traits is shaped by the environment (Knopik et al., 2017). But the role of the environment in mental disorders is accounted for not by risk factors shared by siblings raised in the same family, but by experiences that are unique to individuals. This "nonshared environment" has many sources. Some reflect the influence of forces outside the family, such as peer groups and schools (Harris, 1998). Others reflect relatively random life events, both inside and outside the family, as well as prenatal factors in development (Plomin, 2018).

The strength of heritable factors demonstrated in twin studies contradicts traditional beliefs, especially in PTSD, which has often been considered to be an environmentally driven disorder. For that reason, behavioral genetic research is one of the most important developments in the history of psychology (Plomin et al., 2016). First, it shows that genes have a strong influence on the risk for psychopathology. Second, it contradicts the idea that personality and mental illness are directly and uniquely determined by life experiences. Third, it indicates that the risk for mental illness can be influenced by factors that lie outside the family (and may sometimes be affected by sheer luck).

These findings also help to explain why the effects of trauma are not easily predictable. Adverse events, even highly traumatic ones, do not necessarily lead to PTSD, or to any mental disorder. Instead, psychopathology emerges from interactions between exposure to stressors and vulnerability.

Again, one of the crucial vulnerability factors for PTSD is high trait *Neuroticism*, a temperamental variation leading to more intense emotional reactions to life events. Thus, high Neuroticism describes people who are easily upset by their environment and who have trouble calming down after an emotional reaction. Neuroticism is high in all mental disorders characterized by anxiety and depression (Costa & Widiger, 2015).

Neuroticism is a major domain in one of the best-validated ways to assess personality traits, the Five Factor Model (FFM). These five domains can be remembered by the acronym "OCEAN": Openness (O), Conscientiousness (C), Extraversion (E), Agreeableness (A), and Neuroticism (N). While high levels of N are associated with anxiety and depression, low levels of C and A can be associated with personality disorders. E and O do not, by themselves, have a consistent relationship to psychopathology. The FFM is marked by gender differences: Women are more neurotic, more extraverted, more agreeable, and more conscientious than men (Schmitt et al., 2008; Weisberg et al., 2011).

A meta-analysis found that the heritability of N is about 40% (Vukasović & Bratko, 2015), similar to what we find for traits of all kinds, as well as for PTSD and most other mental disorders. While 40% is less than half the variance, it is sufficient to have a major influence on clinical outcomes.

Research consistently confirms a strong link between N and vulnerability to PTSD. This relationship was first established with the publication of a classical longitudinal Australian study of firefighters (McFarlane, 1988). When N was measured *prior* to exposure, higher levels on that trait predicted who would develop symptoms after life-threatening fires. Previous adverse experiences were also predictive of an outcome of PTSD. The large-scale community surveys in Detroit by Breslau et al. (1991, 1998) found the same relationship in a general population sample.

These findings have been replicated over and over again ever since. But what accounts for them? Both heritable factors and life experiences turn out to be important.

GENES AND SUSCEPTIBILITY TO PTSD

A large body of research shows that genetic vulnerability plays a role in PTSD (Afifi et al., 2010). But we should not think of genetic research as involving the identification of a single gene for a trait or a pathological outcome. Most outcomes in psychology are polygenic, and single genes rarely account for the heritability of any mental disorder. Instead, interactions between hundreds (or thousands) of genes are associated with major psychopathology (Paris, 2020d).

This level of complexity is clearly challenging. *Genome-wide association studies* (GWAS), in which *all* sites on the genome are examined for correlation with an outcome, have been used to assess these effects. It allows for an estimate of a *polygenic risk score* (i.e., the sum of all correlated variants). The GWAS method has been applied to PTSD in a large international community sample (Nievergelt et al., 2019). The results showed that these scores account for somewhere between 5% and 20% of the variance. This result is similar to what has been found in many other mental disorders. GWAS findings parallel those that emerge from behavioral genetics, even if there is still a gap between what polygenic risk scores account for and the higher scores that generally emerge from behavior genetics.

It is now well established that PTSD is itself partially heritable (Stein et al., 2002). The overall heritability of PTSD was estimated in a Canadian study to be 38% (Afifi et al., 2010). An Australian longitudinal twin study (Sartor et al., 2012) found the heritability of PTSD to be 46%. The Environmental Risk Twin Study (E-Risk), which studied a cohort of twins in the United Kingdom who were followed longitudinally from childhood to adulthood (Lewis et al., 2019), may eventually report heritability for PTSD but has not done so yet.

Notably, in a sample of veterans, *each one* of the PTSD symptoms listed in the third edition of the *Diagnostic and Statistical Manual of Mental Disorders* (DSM-III; American Psychiatric Association, 1980) was shown to be separately heritable (at least 30% of outcome) after controlling for combat exposure (True et al., 1993). Of some interest, in the same sample, Lyons et al. (1993) found that combat exposure itself was moderately heritable, possibly because of genetic variations affecting risk-taking behaviors.

In summary, the genetic factors that affect the susceptibility to PTSD are largely reflected in levels of N, which interact with previous exposures to produce individual differences in vulnerability to traumatic events.

NEUROSCIENCE AND PTSD

A good deal of neuroscience research has examined the biological effects of trauma. Many of these studies focused on the hypothalamic–pituitary–adrenal (HPA) axis (Dunlop & Wong, 2019). This pathway links the brain to the endocrine system, specifically to the production of cortisol. Research suggests that PTSD patients suffer from elevated activity in the HPA axis, leading to a failure to moderate stress responses (Yehuda, 2002). But since the HPA axis is not a simple pathway, consistent relationships are not always found (Speer et al., 2019).

Another possible mechanism involves epigenetics. These are the switches than can change the activity of genes in response to environmental conditions (O'Donnell & Meaney, 2020). These environmentally triggered changes to gene activity do not depend on the sequence of DNA. For example, many findings have described abnormalities in the HPA axis, a system that determines stress responses (Lanius & Olff, 2017). Thus, multiple adversities could, through effects on genetic switches, regulate the HPA system to be overreactive to later stressors (Ryan et al., 2016). Daskalakis et al. (2018) suggested that interactions of that kind can help account for individual variations in vulnerability to trauma. To some extent, epigenetic changes can be passed on to the next generation: Children of Holocaust survivors have abnormalities of the HPA axis similar to those that can be measured in their parents (Yehuda & Lehmer, 2018). Interactions between neurobiology and life experiences could therefore reflect epigenetic changes that prime the organism and further increase environmental sensitivity (Sheerin et al., 2017).

The literature on the neurobiology of PTSD has made great use of functional magnetic resonance imaging (fMRI), which allows researchers to identify activity in specific brain regions. However, while fMRI has been a flagship method in neuroscience, it does not always yield data that add to what we know from clinical observation. It is striking to see imaging findings that show what trauma can do to the brain, but every life circumstance has the potential to change neural circuitry—as does psychotherapy (Satel & Lilienfeld, 2013).

Another area of interest in neuroscience concerns differences in the size of brain structures, and whether specific regions are constructed differently in those who develop a disorder than in those who do not. One focus of investigation on PTSD has been the hippocampus, which tends to be smaller in patients with PTSD (Bremner et al., 1995; Yehuda, 2002). Yet decreased hippocampal volume, often thought to be a consequence of exposure to trauma, is much the same in twin pairs (Gilbertson et al., 2002), suggesting that it could be a biological marker for vulnerability. (The hippocampus processes memories, and a smaller one may do so less effectively.)

One point of controversy is whether traumatic experiences can have permanent effects on the brain. A twin study (Pitman et al., 2006) found neuropsychological similarities between those who had been exposed to combat in war and co-twins who had not. This suggests that regional changes in the brain can precede, rather than follow, traumatic exposure.

One mechanism may be epigenetic, in which the cumulative effects of traumatic events can change the dialing up of responses past the point at which neural systems can handle them (Sheerin et al., 2017). Alternatively, some of these changes in brain function may reflect not the effects of trauma but rather a prior vulnerability that increases the risk for PTSD, which can then be triggered by trauma (Horwitz, 2018).

NEUROTICISM, PTSD, AND EVOLUTION

One way to understand the vulnerability to PTSD is through the lens of natural selection. Behavioral traits are inherited when they increase survival of organisms and the passing on of their genes. This does not mean that personality traits need be the same in all individuals (Nesse, 2019). Rather, trait profiles can be understood as alternative strategies whose effectiveness depends on varying environmental conditions (Beck et al., 2015).

N is a trait in which higher levels show that the psychological immune system is more readily triggered. That can be an advantage when real dangers occur: You are more likely to survive threats if you are willing to act quickly and tolerate false-positive perceptions of danger. (An example often given is that it is better to flee a predator that is not there than to ignore one that is actually there.)

People with unusually low N, such as those with psychopathic traits, tend to die young because they take too many risks (Vaurio et al., 2018). Yet low levels of N can be an advantage in situations that call for boldness and rapid response. There are both advantages and disadvantages in these variations, and depending on the environment, they affect vulnerability to trauma.

Once again, an analogy can be made with the immune system. Failure to develop immune responses can be dangerous if not fatal. But in autoimmune diseases, or in the "cytokine storms" that kill some patients with COVID-19, hair-trigger overresponsiveness to stressors can be maladaptive.

These considerations help to explain why personality traits vary so much from one person to another. Different trait profiles work best under different conditions. In a parallel situation in medicine, a genetic predisposition to diabetes will be selected for in populations that live in an environment with uncertain food supplies but selected against in environments, such as our modern world, where food is all too abundant.

In summary, people who are high on N are more susceptible to internalizing disorders that include anxiety and depression, as well as PTSD. They react more strongly to stressors and take longer to calm down.

PREVIOUS EXPOSURE TO TRAUMA

Heritability is not the only reason for individual differences in susceptibility to trauma; another factor is previous exposure. By and large, single events lack the capacity to override the protection of the psychological immune system, but multiple adversities have cumulative effects that eventually trigger symptoms (Breslau et al., 1991; Rutter, 2013). This dose–response relationship has sometimes been called "complex" trauma, to be discussed in Chapter 7.

Prospective longitudinal studies, following cohorts in the community, offer a way to unravel how different people process trauma. This research design avoids the problem of inaccurate retrospective recall of life events. In a systematic review of 54 studies of longitudinal cohorts that examined PTSD as an outcome (DiGangi et al., 2013), many symptoms that patients or clinicians might attribute to a traumatic event were already present prior to exposure. A research program in an American city that followed children who had been assessed in the justice system for well-established histories of abuse over several decades yielded very similar findings (Widom, 1999). As Widom (1999, p. 1223) concluded, "Victims of child abuse (sexual and physical) and neglect are at increased risk for developing PTSD, but childhood victimization is not a sufficient condition. Family, individual, and lifestyle variables also place individuals at risk and contribute to the symptoms of PTSD."

The point is that single risk factors must be viewed in the larger context of a patient's overall life history. The cumulative effects of multiple adversities are much more predictive of the development of mental disorders. It is almost always misleading to see PTSD as the result of a single event.

THE BIOPSYCHOSOCIAL MODEL OF PSYCHOPATHOLOGY

When we don't understand the origins of complex disorders, we may be tempted to adopt simple theories that seem to explain everything. For this reason, psychiatry, which explores the mysteries of brain, mind, and mental illness, has suffered from a tendency to fall victim to fads and fallacies of all kinds (Paris, 2013a). Most of these ideas lead to the development of models in which single risk factors are invoked to account for highly complex phenomena. Yet almost all mental disorders emerge from interactions between many risk factors (Paris, 2020d).

Oversimplification and reductionism have long been problems in biological psychiatry, where researchers have, at various times, proposed that abnormal levels of neurotransmitters, deviations in neural circuitry, or variations of single alleles can explain phenomena as complex as mood disorders, anxiety disorders, and psychoses.

Attempts to reduce complexity have also been a problem for psychosocial theories of etiology, which have, over time, attributed the causes of many mental disorders to risk factors such as bad parenting or traumatic experiences. These ideas have often been used to justify psychotherapies that focus on the past rather than on the present.

To be fair, most of us have trouble getting out of the box of linear thinking. We have not been trained to adopt a sophisticated and multivariate approach to cause and effect.

That is why a biopsychosocial (BPS) model is necessary (Engel, 1980). It describes the etiology of disorders as rooted in interactions among biological, psychological and social risk factors. While the BPS model has been criticized for lack of precision (Ghaemi, 2010), it is not possible to be precise as long as we know so little about the precise pathways to psychopathology. A BPS theory is a good place to begin to think about disorders that do not have linear relationships to risk and that are based on multivariate interactions.

The BPS model also offers some practical advantages for clinicians. Once you approach etiology in terms of complex interactions, you will be less likely to believe that disorders have simple causes, or that they can be cured with simple remedies. You will be less likely to prescribe the latest medication or offer the latest psychological intervention without strong supporting evidence. You will be aware that the causes of mental disorder are enormously complex, and that each domain (biological, psychological, and social) of the BPS model combines risks from a multitude of potential factors, all interacting with each other as well as with risk factors in other domains.

A biopsychosocial model is not just a list of risk factors that can be added up to create a rough theory; it provides the basis for the study of how risks from different domains interact with each other. Let us consider the example of people with high N. They are overly sensitive to their environment. And because they tend to be anxious and pessimistic, they may be more difficult for their parents, as well as for their schools, workplaces, intimate partners, and social networks, to manage.

N can be an advantage when there are real dangers to be avoided in life. But this trait can make people more likely to catastrophize, seeing adverse events, even when less pathogenic, as confirming their bias that the world is a dangerous place. N can be buffered by family and social supports that make those who have these traits feel safer in the world.

APPLYING A BPS MODEL TO PTSD

One can build a biopsychosocial model based on a genetic pre-disposition to PTSD rooted in personality traits, interacting with psychological risks such as previous adversity, as well as social risks such as lack of supports. But since each of these domains belongs to a different research tradition, few have attempted to put all the pieces of the puzzle together. For this reason, a prominent group of PTSD investigators argued years ago for giving priority to gene–environment interactions in research on PTSD (Koenen et al., 2008).

Clinically relevant findings emerge from studies of people in dangerous high-risk occupations. Research studies on firefighters and police officers have allowed researchers to apply prospective methodologies, in which risk factors *prior* to trauma, as well as the severity of exposure to a traumatic event, are measured at baseline. In a classic study of Australian fire fighters, McFarlane (1988) found that over time, the longer PTSD symptoms remained, the less they were accounted for by exposure to trauma and the more they were accounted for by innate predispositions. Vulnerability to PTSD strongly reflected personality traits of N, as well as either a family history or a previous history of mental disorder, each of which reflects a heritable component. Later behavioral genetic studies (e.g., Stein et al., 2002) have replicated these findings.

In these prospective studies, many researchers had expected that the most important risk factor would be the severity of the stressor. That turned out not to be the case. For PTSD, N and preexisting mental disorders were the strongest predictors. Similar findings have been reported for war veterans (Mattson et al., 2018), in Breslau et al.'s (1991, 1998) community studies, and in large clinical samples (Hyer et al., 1994). Ogle et al. (2013) concluded that N increases the risk for PTSD symptoms by magnifying the emotionality, availability, and centrality of traumatic memories.

It is important to conduct prospective studies because if N is measured at the same time as PTSD symptoms, it will be unclear what is cause and what is effect. In a twin sample that was followed prospectively (Kendler & Prescott, 2007), N clearly preceded the development of symptoms. Breslau and Schultz (2013) followed over a thousand people for 10 years and conducted multivariate analyses of outcome; once again, N was the most significant predictor, independent of traumatic exposure. It remains possible that other heritable traits, in interaction with psychosocial risks, could also play a role.

Trait N is a complex domain, and specific facets of this trait have been described (Anxiety, Hostility, Depression, Self-consciousness, Impulsiveness, and Vulnerability; Costa & Widiger, 2015), which can also be measured with tools developed for the FFM. For example, a prospective study of pregnant women (Englehard et al., 2003) found that the aspect of N that was the key predictive factor of later PTSD was a high level of emotional arousal.

One of the major problems affecting research in this area is the fuzziness of the PTSD category. While one can separately measure posttraumatic symptoms, most overlap greatly with mood and anxiety disorders. This helps explain why the presence of depression or anxiety prior to trauma reflects underlying traits rather than independent conditions.

Although heritable traits influence whether or not individuals are susceptible to PTSD, the cumulative effects of multiple psychosocial stressors have the capacity to overwhelm the psychological immune system. However, there is some evidence that one of the predictors of PTSD is the nature of the traumatic event. As we have seen, interpersonal violence, with physical assault or rape, carries the highest risk, and is often stronger than life-threatening events of other kinds (Sareen, 2014). These effects might be partly accounted for by feelings of betrayal associated with intimate partner violence and/or with feelings of violation associated with rape.

Clinicians still need to explain why many victims make such bad choices of intimate partners, and why they come back to the same ones, even after repeated incidents of violence. These mechanisms lie well beyond the effects of trauma, and they lead us into the realm of personality. It is well known that traumatic experiences in childhood and adulthood are common in borderline personality disorder, a condition marked by emotion dysregulation and impulsivity. However, this relationship is not specific to any personality profile. Allen et al. (2019) found that avoidant traits, reflecting temperamental anxiety, are also associated with a high risk of PTSD.

To build a BPS model, we also need to invoke a social perspective. The role of social networks in PTSD has not always been recognized. Yet a body of literature points to the importance of emotional support after trauma. Several studies have shown that emotional neglect from significant others, associated with a failure to support those who have endured trauma, can be at least as pathogenic as trauma itself (Stoltenborgh et al., 2013).

We also need to consider the effects of historical and cultural change. PTSD has become more common over time in developed countries, where trauma is less frequent, but the condition remains less common in the developing world, where trauma is more frequent (Duckers & Brewin, 2016). This seems to be a paradox, but explanations could lie in differences in recognition of the syndrome, cultural expectations about trauma, or levels of social support after exposure. Or, as Young (1995) has suggested, PTSD could be a social construct that has a different meaning in societies where traumatic events are not considered unusual.

Finally, it needs to be kept in mind that behavioral genetics shows that about half of the variance affecting PTSD is environmental. All kinds of life events contribute to overall risk. One extra trauma can be the proverbial straw breaking the camel's back.

CORRELATION AND CAUSATION

Mental health professionals are trained to take a careful life history to identify possible risk factors for mental disorders, particularly adverse life experiences. However, these relationships are only *correlations*. It is all too easy to reach unjustified conclusions about whether any risk factor is a *cause* of a mental disorder. This caveat applies equally well to life experiences as to biological variations.

Why is this so? Obviously, correlation is *not* causation. While that is a scientific cliché, it needs to be repeatedly kept in mind to avoid our human tendency to mistakenly "connect the dots." The presence of any risk factor, even when found in the majority of patients with a given disorder, does not mean that it should be seen, by itself, as a causal agent. The human mind is programmed to search for patterns, and it tends toward a linear view of cause and effect (Shermer, 2011). But that is not the way the world works, particularly in human psychology.

Every phenomenon we observe in clinical practice has multiple determinants that interact in a complex way. Mental disorders almost always arise from interactions between multiple genes and multiple environmental effects (Kendler & Prescott, 2007). Unfortunately, clinicians are not trained to think in that way.

Second, clinical inference suffers from biases. One of the most common is an *availability bias* (Kahnemann, 2011). This means that whatever comes most easily to mind tends to be given undue weight. The more dramatic is an adversity, the more likely it is to stand out in our minds, and to be used to account for symptoms.

Clinical inferences also suffer from a *confirmation bias* (Kahnemann, 2011). We do not approach patients with a blank slate. If clinicians are already convinced that a particular risk factor is crucial, they will search for it and focus on its role.

Even though research methods are much more systematic than clinical observations, these biases can still affect the choice of what to measure, as well as the interpretation of data. Most psychological research tests hypotheses that an independent variable is associated with (or is a cause of) changes in a dependent variable. Standard statistical methods require a p-value of less than .05—that is, a 95% chance of finding the same result in a similar sample.

But that is too low a bar. All too many studies in psychology and medicine turn out not to be replicable (Ioannidis, 2005). There are many reasons for this "replication crisis," but one is that a single independent variable, even if its relationship to a dependent variable can be shown to be less than $p = .05$, rarely accounts for a large percentage of the variance of a dependent variable. In other words, single risk factors are only part of a larger complex network of causality, and very complex interactions are required to produce a disorder like PTSD (McNally, 2017).

We can see this problem in genetic studies of mental disorders, where the search for a single gene, or just a few genes, that could account for psychopathology has been largely fruitless. Even when single genes are significantly related to a disorder, they usually account for about 1% of the outcome variance (Paris, 2020d). Even GWAS findings, which amass samples in the thousands to study every variation in alleles, and can add up effects of multiple genes to yield a polygenic risk score, account for only a small percentage of the outcome. The reason is that genetic effects cannot be reduced to the effects of a few genes; rather; they involve highly complex interactions between multiple sites, both coding and non-coding alleles that regulate other genes. Moreover, genetic differences can have different effects in different environments.

The search for specific genes associated with risk has not thus far been successful. In a large-scale GWAS, Duncan et al. (2018) found a heritable component associated with PTSD (25% overall, but about 50% in women), but these heritable risks were shared with other major psychiatric disorders. This suggests that even though vulnerability to PTSD reflects genetic variation, there are no specific genes for the disorder. Much the same picture has been reported for psychosis, depression, and other major categories (Paris, 2020d). As many others have pointed out, genes don't read the DSM. Instead, they influence broader traits that underlie symptoms.

The same problems arise in research on environmental effects. A single risk factor can have a statistically significant relationship to an outcome without accounting for much of the variance. This is the reason why some psychologists have argued that we should stop using p-values and replace them with a measure of *effect size*, which provides a quantitative result in terms of a standard deviation

(Cohen, 1994). Findings that reach p < .05 may still have a small effect size. This statistical standard need not be a yes/no, but rather a score that gives you what has been called "Cohen's d," which can be rated as small (0.2), medium (0.5), or large (0.8).

A deeper problem lies with research methods that only measure selected independent variables. Researchers now have statistical methods based on multiple regression, hierarchical linear modeling, or path analysis—all of which allow them to measure many independent variables to see how much each *separately* relates to either one or multiple dependent variables. But the more variables you measure, the larger your sample needs to be. Researchers are forced to choose. And that leaves the question of bias: whether the choice of potential predictors is sufficiently broad, or whether what has *not* been measured may actually be just as important or more important than what was actually measured.

Most research on psychopathology is based on group differences between samples, which are usually preselected in other respects for homogeneity. Yet causation cannot always be proven when only group differences are considered. Research in psychology often fails to address the need to account for *individual differences* in outcome. And, in the case of PTSD, these differences do not necessarily lie with stressors alone but rather in variation between people in their ability to cope with their environment.

Research showing that people who develop PTSD have predisposing traits that are present prior to exposure to trauma has yielded consistent findings over many decades (Breslau et al., 1991; Yehuda & McFarlane, 1995). Yet these prior risk factors tend to remain unknown to psychotherapists. If clinicians were more aware of this research, they might be less inclined to attribute a wide range of symptoms to adverse life experiences and to diagnose all patients who have a traumatic history with PTSD.

All these biases can lead to an overdiagnosis of PTSD. It is only one of several diagnostic fads that currently afflict psychiatry: The others are bipolar disorder, autistic spectrum disorder, and attention-deficit/hyperactivity disorder (Paris, 2020c). Overdiagnosis reflects, in part, the wish of psychotherapists to listen to and sympathize with their patients' life histories. And ironically, like the dubious concept of "chemical imbalances" in psychiatry, an emphasis on the environment offers a point of view that places responsibility not on patients, but on forces beyond their control.

Chapter 3

Trauma in Historical and Social Perspective

Classifications of mental disorders are not written in stone. Moreover, current diagnoses lack the biomarkers that are used to identify medical conditions. Instead, diagnostic categories describe clusters of symptoms defining characteristic clinical pictures that may or may not correspond to etiological pathways. Posttraumatic stress disorder (PTSD) is not an exception. This chapter will show that ideas about this disorder have changed over time and can be different in different societies.

The construct of PTSD, with its focus on the damaging impact of traumatic events, may be an idea that reflects features of the modern world (Young, 1995). Summerfield (2001) noted that PTSD had "totemic" status because it seems to validate of experiences of suffering. Andreasen (1995) archly commented that PTSD may be the one mental disorder that patients actually want to have. Furedi (2004) argued that recent levels of interest in PTSD are part of a social movement in which psychotherapy itself has earned a unique status in Western culture.

Trauma and posttraumatic symptoms have been viewed differently across the course of recorded history, as well as across societies and cultures. Yet some of the mechanisms leading to PTSD and anxiety disorders may be universal. On an evolutionary level, fearing and avoiding danger, once encountered, is an adaptive strategy (Nesse, 2019). But not everyone processes threats in the same way. And when people lack support from social networks and communities to deal with environmental adversity, one can speak of social risk factors that increase the risk for disorder.

HISTORICAL PERSPECTIVES

PTSD is a relatively new diagnosis that only entered the standard classification of mental disorders a little more than 40 years ago. In the 19th century, interest in the effects of trauma focused on observations about victims of rail accidents or war. Physicians who diagnosed soldiers as suffering from "war neuroses" in the past did not necessarily describe all the same symptoms listed in current diagnostic manuals (Jones & Wessely, 2005). Moreover, psychiatrists of that era could not have imagined a world in which PTSD would be considered to be common, if not ubiquitous, in clinical and community populations.

Studies of PTSD after a war provide a historical perspective (Horwitz, 2018). In the American Civil War, physicians observed what they called "soldier's heart," characterized by fatigue, shortness of breath, palpitations, sweating, and chest pain—more or less the symptoms of what we now call panic attacks. Shortly after the war, clinicians observed "railway spine"—undiagnosable back pain after train accidents. In the First World War, the term "shell shock" reflected a theory that the physical effects of bombardment led to a syndrome marked by fatigue, tremor, confusion, nightmares, and exaggerated reactions to loud noises. In the Second World War, a diagnosis of "combat stress reaction" described a picture of fatigue, apathy, and slowing down of mental processes after exposure to combat. In the first edition of the *Diagnostic and Statistical Manual of Mental Disorders* (DSM-I; American Psychiatric Association, 1952), the term "gross stress reaction" was introduced, but it was dropped in DSM-II (American Psychiatric Association, 1968), which lacked a specific category for this clinical picture.

To a surprising extent, posttraumatic symptoms in each era can be different. McNally (2012) observes that it is hard to find the symptoms of the past in present-day PTSD patients and that it is also hard to find today's symptoms in descriptions form the past. For example, one can find no description in previous wars of soldiers experiencing flashbacks, a central symptom reported by PTSD patients after combat in the Vietnam War (Horwitz, 2018). Careful studies based on British military records have shown that symptoms related to combat exposure have greatly changed over time and that they do not resemble the flashbacks described by Vietnam veterans (Jones et al., 2002; Jones & Wessely, 2005). Survivors of other kinds of trauma, such as the genocide in Cambodia (Hinton & Good, 2015), tend to present a symptomatic pattern marked by more prominent somatic symptoms, which is generally more common in developing nations for internalizing disorders such as depression and anxiety.

PTSD was accepted into DSM-III (American Psychiatric Association, 1980) largely because of the Vietnam War, so that adoption of the diagnosis was as much political as scientific. The impetus came from psychiatrists (especially Chaim Shatan and Robert Lifton) who were opposed to that war. By emphasizing that combat could cause psychological symptoms, even years after exposure, they aimed to strengthen the argument for ending the conflict (Scott, 1990).

The acceptance of PTSD in DSM manuals over the last 40 years has encouraged the expansion of this construct outside military settings. The latter decades of the 20th century marked an era in which sympathy for people who suffer trauma began to have an effect on diagnostic practices. Thus, the PTSD diagnosis was applied to a range of adverse experiences, such as rape, physical violence, natural disasters, and terrorism. In the early decades of the new century, the concept of PTSD was even further expanded, to include responses to insensitive comments that have been called "micro-aggressions." As Horwitz (2018, p. 2) comments:

> As recently as 1980, the sorts of event that were considered to be "traumas" were limited to extreme stressors such as military combat, rape, severe assault, and natural or man-made disasters. Since that time, the range of traumas has expanded to include hearing hate speech, learning of a relative's death, or watching a catastrophe unfold on television. Virtually the entire population experiences such "traumas" during their lifetimes. . . . .
>
> Western, and, increasingly, most cultures now routinely assume that people who are exposed to traumas will develop serious and recurrent negative psychological consequences. Mental health specialists often predict that a pandemic of traumatic psychic conditions will arise after man-made and natural disasters. As a result, trauma counselors have become entrenched in schools, work organizations, hospitals, and police and fire departments to deal with the expected psychological results of disturbing experiences. At the extreme, some instructors in colleges and universities use "trigger warnings" on reading material they feel might precipitate PTSD among their students.

These critiques of the supposed sensitivity of students to minor "traumas," or to poorly chosen words by university teachers, have been made by other social scientists and are associated with the idea that young people today are being coddled, making them less prepared for adult life (Lukianoff & Haidt, 2018). The older idea in Western culture that toughness in the face of adverse or traumatic life events is a virtue seems to have lost purchase.

Another historical change, noted by McNally (2012), is that witnessing violence was not actually considered to be a trauma in the past. Public executions once attracted large groups of spectators who enjoyed observing torture and death. It is also doubtful if people who witnessed public lynching in the American South developed PTSD after doing so. The disappearance of such events was described by Pinker (2019) as one of the triumphs of humanism and the Enlightenment, and that view is now almost universally held.

Some social critics have thought that modern life is associated with higher levels of trauma, which has created a "mental health crisis." A good example is the claim that university students, an unusually talented and fortunate population, seem to be at increasing risk for psychopathology (Duffy et al., 2019). Since I worked part-time at a university health service for 25 years and saw a great range of cases, I find this hard to believe. And research evidence does not support such a conclusion: Rates of mental disorder are generally *lower* in university students than in their peers (Wiens et al., 2020). What is probably happening is that students who are privileged and highly educated are more likely to identify distress and seek treatment for it. Their expectations are high, and they are easily disappointed. They may experience more symptoms without a change in the prevalence of diagnosable disorders.

Yet, over the course of history, most aspects of life have become safer and more predictable (Pinker, 2012). Thus, in spite of a higher level of *reporting* of psychological symptoms, traumatic events themselves have not been shown to be less common than in the past. In fact, the contrary is the case. Moreover, those who insist that problems such as PTSD are increasing may be promoting an agenda to show that modern society is bad and needs to change. Or, as Pinker (2019) wittily noted, some political progressives are so set on changing the world that they hate progress and prefer to deny its existence.

If there *is* a crisis in mental health, it does not derive from an increased prevalence of disorders, but from a combination of increased demand for treatment and longstanding problems with the accessibility of services (Chiu et al., 2020; Kessler et al., 2005b). If people living in modern society are less prepared to deal with trauma, it could be because they regard it as something unusual. This would not have been the case in the past when life was both more brutal and shorter.

However, it is possible that accessibility of social support after trauma has been compromised by the rise of individualism and a decline of collectivism (Markus & Kitayama, 1991). Henrich (2020) points out that individualist values define the psychology of people living in the most developed countries, but these values are much weaker in those living in more traditional societies that define identity in terms of the family and collectivism. Support for this hypothesis has emerged from transcultural studies of PTSD (Kirmayer et al., 2007).

Some data suggest that advanced technology, such as increases in screen time among adolescents, may have negative psychological effects on mental health (Twenge et al., 2018). However, this correlation may not prove causation, and other studies, particularly longitudinal data, have not replicated it (Coyne et al., 2019). By and large, social change tends to produce different forms of psychological symptoms rather than an overall increase (Shorter, 1997).

In short, the data are not consistent with a mental health epidemic among young people. Instead, what we know is that more people are seeking mental health treatment, and that the majority of these additional patients suffer from less severe forms of psychopathology (Olfson et al., 2019).

Another source of the perception of a mental health crisis is that the scope of diagnoses in psychiatry has a tendency to expand with time (Frances, 2013; Paris, 2020c). Shy people may be seen as suffering from social phobia, braggarts may be labeled as narcissistic, and highly introverted people may be seen as falling on an autistic spectrum. Yet those who are overly sensitive to stress are not necessarily candidates for developing a diagnosis of PTSD.

As McNally (2015, p. 47) notes:

A mildly stressful event in a relatively stress-free, comfortable life may produce a more pronounced negative response than a moderately stressful event occurring against a background of marked adversity. If this hypothesis turns out to be true, then public health efforts that increase the safety of communities may fail to reduce the burden of PTSD in society.

Overdiagnosis in psychiatry and clinical psychology can be based on "concept creep," the extension of a construct to more and more phenomena over time (Haslam, 2016). This is a problem affecting all of the mental health professions. Concept creep is much the same mechanism that led Young (1995) to describe PTSD as a "social construct." McNally (2015), in a commentary titled "The Expanding Empire of Psychopathology: The Case of PTSD," described how our view of what is and what is not traumatic has greatly changed over time, and how minor events can be recalibrated as dangerous. As McNally notes (2015, p. 47), "Civilians who underwent the terror of World War II . . . would surely be puzzled to learn that giving birth to a healthy baby after an uncomplicated delivery or encountering obnoxious jokes at work can cause PTSD."

SOCIOCULTURAL PERSPECTIVES

Above and beyond historical change, societies and cultures can and do differ in rates of exposure to trauma and in the prevalence of PTSD. Cross-national differences were found by the World Health Organization (WHO) World Mental Health Survey, which examined the prevalence of traumatic events and PTSD in 24 countries (Benjet et al., 2016; Bromet et al., 2018; Kessler et al., 2017). About 70% of people around the world reported lifetime trauma of some kind; the most common examples were witnessing death or serious injury; experiencing the unexpected death of a loved one; being in a robbery or a life-threatening automobile accident; and experiencing a life-threatening illness or injury. Many of these experiences are a normal part of the human condition, and it is hard to think of anyone who has not had to face at least one of them. In contrast, the original formulation that led to the definition in DSM-III was that traumas leading to PTSD are either unusually severe or repetitive and cumulative.

While there were notable differences in the prevalence of PTSD across countries, the overall risk of disorder after exposure to trauma in the WHO study was only 4%. The prevalence of traumas most likely to lead to PTSD was found to be similar across the globe. The most pathogenic events, in terms of conditional risk for PTSD, were rape (19.0%), intimate partner sexual violence (11.4%), physical abuse by a partner (11.7%), kidnapping (11.0%), and sexual assault other than rape (10.5%). While the WHO study found that PTSD can be recognized all across the world, its precise prevalence depends on whether a broad or narrow definition of the disorder is used. The survey also confirmed the finding that previous trauma, and either a personal history or family history of anxiety disorders, increased risk. But the main limitation of its cross-sectional method was that it described correlations that may or may not be causal.

In a study carried out in 11 European countries (Burri & Maercker, 2014), the same patterns of trauma were associated with PTSD, with most cases derived either from war or from crime, and overall rates of the disorder were correlated with the frequency of these events in the population. The rates across countries were variable, ranging from a prevalence of 6.7% to 4.5%, with the highest rates occurring in countries that had experienced war. While the overall prevalence of PTSD was low, this study was unique in showing that living in countries with low crime rates and a high modern-value orientation predicts a higher PTSD prevalence. These findings might support the hypothesis that modernity, in spite of all its benefits, can be a risk factor for PTSD. As people become more individualistic, they have less access to social supports (Henrich, 2020). These findings might also be consistent with the possibility that when trauma is less common and occurs more unexpectedly, PTSD becomes more likely.

The cross-national and ethnic differences between developed countries in the prevalence of PTSD point to the importance of whether societies retain traditional values or adopt modern values. Maintaining tradition is associated with conformity, benevolence, and a reverence for customs, while modernity is linked to achievement, hedonism, and a desire for stimulation (Paris,

2013b). Traditional societies provide strong social support as long as one conforms to their point of view on the world, but they are relatively intolerant of choices based on individual needs. In contrast, modern societies require people to build their own social networks, which some people are better at than others. And those who lack strong social supports may be more likely to develop chronic symptoms.

However, belonging to a traditional society may not always be protective. Schwartz (1994) developed a system designed to assess social values. Applying this measure, Maercker et al. (2011) found that Chinese crime victims who espoused traditional values were more likely than German victims to develop PTSD and to have more severe symptoms. Thus, these findings do not support the idea that PTSD is entirely modern, and they may point to an inflexibility in some traditional societies that may impede social support. Perhaps the results would have been different if the comparison group to Germans had not been Chinese.

Yet in the WHO survey (Kessler et al., 2017), the highest rates of the disorder were found in Western countries. Duckers and Brewin (2016) noted a "vulnerability paradox" in that PTSD is much more common in highly developed countries than in those afflicted by widespread poverty. McNally (2018) suggested that the paradox could be resolved if PTSD is more frequent in subpopulations within wealthier countries who are more vulnerable. It is also possible that the culture of highly developed countries creates different expectations about how much adversity is normal. Thus, people growing up in more affluent settings could have a lower level of psychological immunity to trauma. Some years ago, I asked a physician who was conducting research in Ethiopia during a major famine whether she had seen PTSD in the survivors. Her answer was "they were too busy for that."

Social support reduces the risk for mental disorders of all kinds (Ozbay et al., 2007). That is also the case for PTSD (Wagner et al., 2016). But social support may not correlate necessarily with whether societies are traditional or modern; trauma victims may receive less social support because of values favoring family loyalty and avoiding loss of face. Thus, PTSD may not present in the same way in people from strongly traditional cultures. Instead of reporting psychological symptoms, distress may be communicated through somatic channels (Kramer et al., 2002). People in Asian societies, such as survivors of the Cambodian genocide, rarely report avoidance or numbing but describe more somatic complaints (Hinton & Lewis-Fernandez, 2011). The same tendency to somatization can be seen in cultures that do not attribute distress to concepts such as anxiety or depression. Thus, while PTSD may be universal in some form, its present definition makes it into a culture-bound disorder. The DSM criteria for the disorder do not fully reflect the range of symptoms seen in non-Western cultures, or in subcultures within developed societies.

Moreover, the benefits of modernity can work against us when it comes to trauma. McNally nicely summarizes this issue as follows (2018, pp. 129–130):

Perhaps one unfortunate consequence of the otherwise undeniable benefits of modernity is diminished resilience. Our relatively greater comfort, safety, health, and well-being may have rendered us more vulnerable to stressors far less toxic than the ones occurring during World War II, for example. If so, then the decline in violence occurring over the past thousand years, the mid-twentieth century notwithstanding . . . , may have only broadened the kinds of stressors that can incite PTSD rather than diminishing its incidence over time.

PTSD AND THE CULTURE OF TRAUMA

The diagnosis of PTSD may be partly shaped by what has been called a "culture of trauma" (McNally, 2015). The disorder may be a social construct but is socially useful in that it legitimizes the suffering of those who have been victimized (Summerfield, 2001). Young (1995), an anthropologist who studied PTSD in a Veterans Administration Hospital, described PTSD as follows:

> The disorder is not timeless, nor does it possess an intrinsic unity. Rather, it is glued together by the practices, technologies, and narratives with which it is diagnosed, studied, treated, and represented and by the various interests, institutions, and moral arguments that mobilized these efforts and resources . . . traumatic memory is a man-made object. It originates in the scientific and clinical discourses of the nineteenth century; before that time, there is unhappiness, despair, and disturbing recollections, but no traumatic memory, in the sense that we know it today.

As we have seen, PTSD does not take the same symptomatic form in all historical periods, and there are historical differences in what is defined as a trauma. Moreover, responses to trauma can be expressed in other ways than DSM-5 or ICD-11 criteria. Features now considered central, such as flashbacks, were almost never reported in British soldiers prior to the Gulf War of 1991; instead, feelings of weakness, somatic symptoms, and anxiety and depression were the most common complaints in past wars (Jones & Wessely, 2005). Finally, cultural expectations shape the symptoms of PTSD and the likelihood of its development after adverse events (Hinton & Good, 2015).

In short, PTSD is a heterogeneous construct, not a distinct disorder (Young & Breslau, 2016). In many ways, the diagnosis reflects a modern world that has adopted what might be called a "culture of trauma" (Alford, 2016). In some ways, suffering has been fetishized while adverse life events are seen as the key drivers of human misery. This point of view may be at least partly true. But that way of thinking does not take into account variations in susceptibility to trauma, the cumulative effects of earlier experiences, and a society that encourages people to define themselves as suffering from PTSD, allowing them to feel victimized as well as entitled to compensation, either financially or in the form of therapy (Young, 1995). Some of these patients meet criteria for a comorbid diagnosis of personality disorder (Paris, 2020a). If every problem is attributed to a past traumatic event, evidence-based specialized treatment for overlapping conditions may be not be offered, and every intervention will be "trauma-focused."

THE MYTH OF TRIGGER WARNINGS

The concept of a "trigger warning" is to alert people about exposure to potentially distressing ideas or facts (Bellet et al., 2018). These warnings have been widely applied in universities, where they have been used to prepare students for exposure to material that might upset them—or to justify cancelling invitations to controversial speakers. These practices are based on the idea that so many people have been traumatized that they should be protected from retraumatization. However, some writers believe that trigger warnings hamper free academic inquiry, and they can reduce resilience by sheltering students (Lukianoff & Haidt, 2018). Moreover, encouraging avoidance of cues to trauma runs counter to key mechanisms of therapy for PTSD and, by reinforcing an identity linked to being a victim of trauma, may therefore be counterproductive in the long term (McNally, 2007). As Bellet et al. (2018, p. 131) argue:

> Trigger warnings suggest that trauma survivors will have difficulty with content encountered in daily life, and may lead people to believe that they are likely to develop PTSD should they encounter trauma, causing them to iatrogenically catastrophize acute posttraumatic symptoms. Further, receiving constant reminders of potential emotional harm may contribute to perceptions of heightened vulnerability, fostering a maladaptive self-identification as a victim. Similarly, trigger warnings may also change the way that people think about others' vulnerability in the wake of trauma. Trigger warnings may raise awareness of the difficulties of people suffering from PTSD. However, they may also create the impression that the experience of trauma always renders survivors emotionally incapacitated. In reality, most trauma survivors are resilient and show few symptoms of PTSD after an initial period of adjustment. The perception of trauma survivors as dysregulated victims may contribute to negative stigma concerning the very individuals trigger warnings are intended to protect.

This social trend is a good example of how well-meaning ideas about trauma can turn out to be counterproductive in the long run. There is an analogy here to infectious diseases in modern societies. Ultimately, exposure to upsetting words or actions is not preventable. It follows that we are better off providing some degree of exposure, a kind of "vaccination" against trauma, while offering people the tools to deal with adversity.

POLITICS, IDENTITY, AND TRAUMA

Trauma is an emotional issue and is also a political problem. One underlying issue is whether adverse experiences can be eliminated by reforming society, or whether trauma is part of the human condition and can at best be minimized. Pinker (2012) describes these two points of views as a utopian vision versus a tragic vision of human nature. They are associated either with political liberalism or conservatism. Yet today's society is now much less violent, promotes more liberty, and is more rational than in the past. A vast body of evidence supporting these conclusions has been reviewed by Pinker (2019). For example, children are less likely to be abused today, either by their peers or by their own families, and adults are less likely to be murdered. Yet people who stand on the left of the political spectrum, and who adhere to a utopian vision, are not satisfied with the current level of social progress, pointing to continued and serious inequities. That may be why they tend to be resistant to the idea that progress is real—for fear of letting their guard down against injustice. To be fair, some pessimistic philosophers on other points of the political spectrum (e.g., Gray, 2013) have also expressed skepticism about making the world better, arguing that human progress is largely an illusion. Those on the right, and who adhere to a tragic vision, tend to have an individualistic perspective and are dubious about the value of social interventions. As Haidt (2012) has demonstrated, the two sides of the spectrum also differ because they do not begin with the same values and they prioritize them differently.

These different points of view have affected debates about the impact of trauma. Anyone who puts an emphasis on individual vulnerability can be accused of "blaming the victim," or of a failure to believe narratives of victimization. Yet the fact that most people are resilient to trauma, while others are more vulnerable, remains an uncomfortable truth for some but provides realistic hope for others.

The idea that trauma can be incorporated into one's individual identity is important for understanding the importance of a PTSD diagnosis in contemporary life (Berman et al., 2020) It is also associated with greater severity of PTSD symptoms (Berntsen & Rubin, 2007), which could either mean that those with a more severe disorder see their suffering as more central, or that developing an identity as a victim of trauma works against recovery. Conversely, there is evidence that posttraumatic growth can sometimes lead to the formation of a more stable social identity (Muldoon et al., 2019).

In summary, PTSD has become a central concern for contemporary society. Its use by clinicians to account for all kinds of complex psychopathological phenomena has spread to the culture at large. It remains to be determined whether this is a positive or a negative development.

Chapter 4

Risk, Resilience, and Trauma

THE UBIQUITY OF RESILIENCE

Risk refers to the statistical probability that an individual will develop a mental disorder—even if most people at risk never develop one. *Resilience* refers, literally, to the ability to "bounce back" from the impact of adverse life events without developing psychological symptoms.

We might think of resilience as a defense system against psychological trauma. Being able to move past trauma is not just a matter of luck; it depends on capacities intrinsic to the individual that can be termed a psychological immune system (Gilbert et al., 1998). Just as immunological mechanisms protect us against the physical attack of microorganisms, resilience protects us against the emotional effects of adverse life events.

Research supports a general principle, based on a very large body of research (Rutter et al., 2012), that resilience to adversity is the norm, not the exception. This conclusion is consistent with the principles of evolutionary psychology (Buss, 2005). Adversity in the course of life is inevitable, and those who cannot deal with such events will be less likely to survive and bear children of their own. If resilience were not ubiquitous, people would be more vulnerable and less likely to reproduce. Natural selection therefore favors the development of innate protective mechanisms against stressful events.

But what determines whether people are resilient or vulnerable? Based on the research reviewed in Chapter 2, we can safely assume that the capacity for resilience is partially heritable. But what exactly is inherited, and how does the environment promote psychological immunity?

INDIVIDUAL DIFFERENCES IN RESILIENCE

The environment in which the human species evolved was dangerous. In the famous phrase of the English philosopher Thomas Hobbes, it could be described as "nasty, brutish, and short." In hunter-gatherer societies, starvation was never far away, predation was a real risk, strangers were often physically dangerous, and life-threatening diseases were endemic (Pinker, 2012). It is therefore not surprising that people often died young and that many children did not live to be adults.

In short, traumatic events in prehistory were much more common than they are today. Since humans are characterized by an unusually long childhood that allows them to learn the complex tasks required of an adult, they need to be born with an ability to learn. The acquisition of new skills plays an important role in helping us to rise above adversity.

Resilience, like any other mental capacity or trait, varies between individuals. The effects of trauma depend on how the mind assimilates and processes adverse life events. Personality traits, rooted in temperament, are a crucial element of a system designed to deal with environmental challenges (Beck et al., 2015). In other words, the outcome of trauma depends on both nature and nurture, involving *gene–environment interactions*.

These pathways depend a good deal on individual differences in personality. Some people have personality profiles that make them more sensitive to trauma, and they react badly to adverse events. Those who have traits that make them *less* sensitive to the environment will be more immune to stressful experiences, and some may even show what has been called "steeling"—that is, greater resilience after trauma (Rutter et al., 2012). Most people lie on a continuum between these extremes, allowing adaptation to normative levels of adversity. Research also shows that trauma does not necessarily affect children more severely than adults. For example, a 40-year follow-up of child survivors of the Holocaust found that children who survived this severely traumatic experience were more resilient than adult survivors (Sigal & Weinfeld, 2001).

In fact, children need to be tougher than adults. Researchers who have conducted long-term follow-up studies have been surprised to observe that problems in childhood, such as serious family conflicts, often prove to have few long-term effects (Kagan, 1994). Clinicians find this hard to understand because most of the patients they see are less resilient than those who do not come for treatment. They get the incorrect impression that trauma causes inevitable and serious damage to all who are exposed. But the patients clinicians see are those who are more susceptible to the environment and who have more trouble getting past adversities.

It is better to have a happy childhood than an unhappy one, but statistical associations cannot be used to make accurate predictions of adult outcomes. Many people develop mental disorders in spite of a happy childhood, and many people with an unhappy childhood function well in adulthood (Kagan, 1998). One can be misled by research showing relationships between trauma and later symptoms, which may be driven by a subgroup of vulnerable individuals, even if most do not suffer the same sequelae. This is just another example of how correlation does not prove causation.

The situation is different when adversities are multiple, start early, and remain in place for years on end, leading to *cumulative* effects (Rutter et al., 2012). Even the strongest psychological immune system can be overloaded and reach a breaking point. Moreover, most of the important adverse events during childhood, such as family discord, parental psychopathology, and low socioeconomic status, are strongly intercorrelated, leading to a cumulative effect of multiple risks (Rutter & Rutter, 1993). For this reason, it is a mistake to isolate adverse events and to fail to take into account the contexts that make them more harmful.

TRAUMA AND RESILIENCE

Psychological models of development, which emphasize the influence of the past on the present, have had an important influence on the practice of psychotherapy. One of these, whose history goes back for over a century, is Freud's view that adult symptoms are largely the outcome of early childhood experiences. A related idea that seems to be particularly popular today is that traumatic experiences at any age tend to be the cause of symptoms of all kinds (Kagan, 1998).

It is true that a large body of research shows that adversities during childhood, particularly when severe, are a risk factor for a wide range of mental disorders, including major depression (Lippard & Nemeroff, 2020). Yet an equally large body of studies, particularly those using a prospective design in community samples, show that only a minority of those exposed to childhood trauma develop mental disorders in adulthood (Fergusson et al., 2008, 2011).

This contradiction can be readily resolved. Trauma lowers *thresholds* for psychopathology but does not consistently predict outcomes; there are just too many exceptions. Moreover, clinicians do not usually see people who grow up to become well-functioning adults in spite of adversity in childhood. They do see people who have experienced few serious life adversities and who still develop mental disorders, even if these cases do not always make an impression on their thinking.

Psychotherapists who only see a limited number of patients in a lifetime get a biased impression of what childhood trauma can do. All patients have stories to tell, and many of these narratives are gripping and poignant. But it is all too tempting to hypothesize links between the past and the present that can be interpreted as causal. Early in my own career, under the influence of my teachers, I became quite adept at this game, making facile "formulations," finding parallels between current symptoms and childhood problems. But my conclusions were little but examples of a confusion between correlation and causation.

Now, over a 50-year career, I have carried out tens of thousands of consultations. However, clinical experience may not make us wiser if we are biased to connect dots that should not be connected. Eventually, exposure to the scientific literature, particularly studies in nonclinical populations, led me to question the strength of the relationship between mental disorders and trauma. Once I got past my bias, avoiding a preference for what is plausible rather than well established, I came to see that the risk factors for mental disorders are almost always complex, multiple, and interactive (Paris, 2020b).

Consider this example from my own research group (Paris, 2020a). A study we conducted of patients with borderline personality disorder (BPD) found that about a third had a significant history of childhood sexual abuse (CSA). Similar findings have emerged from other studies (Zanarini, 2000). The relationship is somewhat stronger if one takes into account parameters of abuse such as the identity of the perpetrator and the duration and severity of the abuse (Browne & Finkelhor, 1986), each of which moderates the outcome. Since the studies that reported the highest rates of trauma had defined it broadly, we were careful to exclude CSA events that were either rare or unlikely to be pathogenic (such as single incidents that did not involve physical contact). In addition, to avoid recovered memories, we only scored events that were clearly recalled. Moreover, a meta-analysis of the effect of CSA on BPD (Fossati et al., 1999) found an overall effect size of .28, which is moderate but not large. This effect size is consistent with the conclusion that CSA is a risk factor for BPD but is neither necessary nor sufficient, by itself, to cause the disorder.

Finally, it is notable that child abuse has been on the decline for many years (Finkelhor & Jones, 2006; Shields et al., 2016, 2019), while the disorders associated with it, such as PTSD and BPD, have not. What research does show is that a history of CSA makes BPD more severe and leads to a worse prognosis (Porter et al., 2020). Our results, in which a history of trauma was not reported in two thirds of the sample, were consistent with research showing high rates of resilience in community populations. In fact, community studies show that only a significant minority of non-patients develop long-term sequelae from CSA, while a majority are resilient (Fergusson et al., 1996a, 1996b; Hailes et al., 2019). These findings reflect the difference between a statistically based *risk factor* and a direct and unique cause.

RISK AND RESILIENCE IN COMMUNITY POPULATIONS

Studies of risk and resilience studies need to avoid the problem of clinical samples that are biased by multiple risk factors and lower levels of resilience. Our understanding can benefit greatly from research on nonclinical populations. The most important projects have followed cohorts of children in the community over time. This longitudinal approach allows for a more precise assessment of resilience.

Community studies have their own limitations: They may not contain a sufficiently large number of individuals who suffered the most serious adversities. For this reason, researchers can choose to follow up high-risk samples, children who have already been identified as being *at risk*. Not all of this research has specifically examined traumatic events, but studies have evaluated the effect of childhood adversity on adult development.

Follow-up Studies of Children in the Community

THE ISLE OF WIGHT STUDY

Decades ago, Rutter conducted a famous study on the Isle of Wight in the United Kingdom (Rutter et al., 1976). The location of the study was no accident, as longitudinal research is better carried out in semirural settings where people do not move around as much as city dwellers. The key finding was that a combination of *cumulative,* but not single, adversities in children was associated with a prevalence of mental disorder that was close to 20%. This is a rather high rate—but 80% of those exposed to the same risk factors did not develop *any* mental disorder.

In general, childhood trauma, even when it involves multiple risks, leads to serious sequelae in about a quarter of those exposed. But to paraphrase a cliché, one can see the cup as three-quarters full rather than one-quarter empty.

THE HAWAII STUDY

In another classic study, Werner and Smith (1992) studied high-risk children who were followed longitudinally and evaluated up to age 30. This cohort was drawn from poverty-stricken Hawaiian plantation workers who were at risk due to poverty and family dysfunction. Yet most of the children in this study, even those exposed to multiple adversities related to dysfunctional families and emotional neglect, became fully competent adults.

What were the characteristics of the minority in Werner's cohort who *did* develop significant pathology? One was a problematic temperament reflecting higher neuroticism and environmental sensitivity. In contrast, personality traits that promoted coping proved to be highly protective against the impact of adversity. More specifically, children who had better social skills, were more intelligent, and were more persistent in mastering tasks did better than those who lacked these characteristics.

Another finding of the Hawaii study was that stressful environmental circumstances were associated with consistent sequelae only in a high-risk subgroup, consisting of 10% of the total cohort. These children suffered from *multiple* adversities, most particularly dysfunction or breakup of the nuclear family, and/or parental mental illness. Once again, the cumulative effects of adversity were demonstrated by a strong relationship between the total number of risk factors and the likelihood of a pathological outcome. Two thirds of children with multiple adversities developed serious difficulties with behavior or mood as adults. Yet, even at this unusually high level of risk, it is notable that another one third of this subgroup became competent adults.

Thus, the Hawaii study confirmed the findings of the Isle of Wight study: Children are most likely to become affected when adversities are multiple and cumulative.

THE ALBANY–SARATOGA STUDY

Cohen et al. (2017) conducted a large-scale longitudinal study of children in two counties in New York State with the aim of determining the predictors of antisocial behavior, substance abuse, and personality disorder. Data were collected over a period of 20 years. The results showed that neither parental death and divorce nor child-rearing practices (such as lack of closeness or punishment) were predictive of these outcomes. The psychosocial risk factors inside the family associated with the most sequelae were parental mental illness and parental sociopathy and, to a lesser extent, remarriage and change of neighborhood. As in the Hawaii study, abuse and neglect raised the risk for psychopathology, but associations were largely accounted for by a severely affected subgroup. In general, social class and school and peer influences were better predictors of delinquency and substance abuse than family dysfunction.

Lifetime Follow-ups of Adolescents

THE GRANT STUDY

This well-known prospective study of Harvard graduates obtained baseline data in the 1930s. Vaillant (2012) later followed this cohort from attendance at university to old age. Although no direct measurements were made about childhood events, the study assessed the quality of recollected childhood experiences. This variable had little or no predictive value for psychological maturity in adulthood. Instead, school performance and defense styles, both of which tend to reflect favorable or unfavorable personality traits, were the best predictors of functioning in later life. There were also no effects of childhood trauma on functioning in old age. But since these subjects all attended Harvard, and since all were men, the sample was in no way representative of the population as a whole.

FOLLOW-UPS OF CHILDREN AND ADOLESCENTS AT RISK

Research on children growing up in urban slums or in rural poverty yields similar findings. An inner-city sample of men who grew up in the 1930s, originally studied by Glueck and Glueck (1950), was followed into adulthood (Snarey & Vaillant, 1985). In contrast to the conventional wisdom that slums must breed crime and disorder, most subjects were socially mobile and grew up to lead productive adult lives.

Another prospective investigation, the Cambridge–Somerville study, was initiated during the Great Depression to predict which inner-city children would become delinquent. When the cohort was followed into adulthood at ages 45 to 53, criminality in adulthood was related to measures of deficient childrearing, often associated with parental alcoholism and criminality (McCord, 1983). Even so, most of the subjects grew out of their earlier behavioral problems and did not become criminals.

A study in Quebec, Canada, was also designed to predict antisocial behavior (Tremblay et al., 2018). It followed cohorts of over 3,000 schoolchildren into adulthood: One group was from the community, and another group was considered to be at high risk for later criminality because of behavior problems. To determine whether antisocial behavior in later life could be predicted, it elaborated on the well-known longitudinal study of Robins (1966), which found that children with conduct disorder were particularly likely to develop these features in adulthood. By now, the research team has published hundreds of scientific papers based on this data. But the project fell victim to a problem that afflicts most longitudinal research: attrition over time, with losses of about 43% of the sample during the adult years. Thus, the more recent findings from this cohort, when subjects were in their 30s, may be less generalizable.

Studies of Institutionalized Children

Children raised in institutions are a particularly high-risk population. This is because they suffer from severe emotional neglect, especially if they are not adopted into a new family. The results of one major study of women who had been reared in institutions early in their childhood demonstrated that while severe adversity was associated with a poorer overall outcome, resilience was more common (Rutter & Quinton, 1984). In women, leaving home in a reasonable and planned way (as opposed to getting pregnant and/or marrying impulsively) was protective, and those who married successfully were eventually indistinguishable from women raised in normal families. The authors suggested that favorable temperamental characteristics, such as higher persistence and lower impulsivity, may have been responsible for resilience in the face of adversity.

The most important study of orphans in recent years examined the long-term outcome of children who had been placed at birth in Romanian orphanages, where they were severely neglected, but who were later adopted by families in the United Kingdom (Rutter et al., 2012). This can be considered to be a "natural experiment," testing whether early deprivation can be compensated for by later experiences. The cohort has now been followed into adulthood. The results of the follow-up are encouraging for most of the children but more discouraging for a more severely affected subgroup. On the one hand, the majority of these children grew up to become asymptomatic adults. However, a subgroup developed significant problems in socialization, such as social disinhibition and what the researchers called "quasi-autism." These outcomes were associated with longer stays in an institution. Thus, when environments are consistently and severely adverse, natural mechanisms of resilience can be overwhelmed.

Birth Cohort Studies

Many researchers have studied the outcome of adversity by obtaining access to large community samples followed from birth. Two of the best-known examples are the British National Longitudinal Study (BNLS), in which all children born in the United Kingdom over a period of several months in 1958 were followed into adulthood, and the National Survey of Health and Development (NSHD), which followed a birth cohort born in 1946 until 1983 (Wadsworth et al., 2006). In both cases, the findings showed that most children who suffered major early adversities eventually did well, while a minority developed symptoms, most often when faced with major stressors in adult life. Depression in adulthood was related to earlier stressors, recent life events, and higher levels of Neuroticism.

We should keep in mind that while many results from these studies have been statistically significant, the cohorts were very large, so that the findings may not apply to *most* people suffering adversity. The results suggest that there is a vulnerable minority who are most affected by life experiences at any stage and who are most likely to develop psychopathology.

A long-term follow-up study into adulthood of a birth cohort in Dunedin, New Zealand, led by Avshalom Caspi and Terri Moffitt, is one of the most important longitudinal studies of children in the present century. Researchers have reported a wealth of data from this cohort (Belsky et al., 2020; Poulton et al., 2015). Its findings have supported etiological theories based on gene–environment interactions. Although prediction was not strong, and there were many exceptions, impulsivity and anxiety as early as age 3 were statistically associated with a risk for adult antisocial behavior (Caspi et al., 1996). This concords with other data showing that the early appearance of impulsivity (Anokhin et al., 2015) and anxiety sensitivity (Stein et al., 1999) have long-term impacts on development. This is probably due to the fact that these temperamental characteristics are heritable, as shown by behavioral genetic research (Knopik et al., 2017). Similar findings have emerged from studies of antisocial behavior (Farrington et al., 1988), in which the strongest factors favoring resilience in high-risk samples were an agreeable temperament, a higher IQ associated with good school performance, and better peer relationships.

The E-Risk Longitudinal Twin Study in the United Kingdom was begun by Caspi and Moffitt in 1998. It differs from other research designs because its sample consists entirely of twins, allowing researchers to separate the effects of genes and environment. The research has been following a group of twins (N = 2,332) from age 5 for over 20 years (Trouton et al., 2002). This study has been particularly interested in the outcome of victimization during adolescence. In a recent report examining self-harm behaviors (Baldwin et al., 2019) the authors summarized their conclusions as follows (p. 536):

> Risk for self-injurious thoughts and behaviors in victimized adolescents is explained only in part by the experience of victimization. Pre-existing vulnerabilities account for a large

proportion of the risk. Therefore, effective interventions to prevent premature death in victimized adolescents should not only target the experience of victimization but also address pre-existing vulnerabilities.

Another focus of interest from the E-Risk Group concerned the presence of "borderline" symptoms—that is, features in adolescence that closely resemble a diagnosis of BPD—and whether they can predict other forms of pathology during the transition to adulthood (Wertz et al., 2020). The finding here was that while BPD symptoms predicted a poor outcome, they were largely driven by genetic rather than environmental factors. This is a good example of how twin samples can yield results that might never have been apparent in cohorts whose genetic vulnerability is not measured.

MECHANISMS OF RESILIENCE

What mechanisms, either genetic or environmental, account for the ability to rise above adversity? I will begin by summarizing the views of Rutter et al. (2012), a research group which has contributed so much to our understanding of resilience.

Rutter notes that research in recent years has come to focus more on resilience that on risk alone. He offers the example of the new field of "positive psychology," which studies what makes people happy, and not just unhappy. He mentions the possibility that low doses of potential trauma (such as short separations from attachment figures) may allow for a steeling effect. (This idea reminds me of how we use vaccines to stimulate the immune system.) Rutter does point out that the now-voluminous research on gene–environment interactions points to important mechanisms behind resilience. Finally, he notes that the life course can be marked by turning points, in which a positive factor (such as an important relationship) comes to cancel out many of the effects of adverse factors.

By and large, personality traits, which are heritable but also influenced by environment, are among the strongest predictors of resilience, with lower levels of Neuroticism being of particular significance (Costa & Widiger, 2015). Research clearly shows that some temperamental qualities are better than others for making the best use of environmental opportunities. Werner and Smith (1992) described them as an attractive personality, intelligence, persistence, a variety of interests, the capacity to be alone, and an optimistic approach to life. People are not passive recipients of external inputs but actively shape their environment to meet their needs.

Accessible social support networks are another important element in resilience. Classic studies of social cohesion help to explain why communities vary in overall levels of psychopathology (Leighton et al., 1963). Social support is particularly important for children with a difficult temperament, who may otherwise have difficulty finding a social niche. Traditional societies, which provide guaranteed social roles for almost everyone, may protect vulnerable children from developing some forms of psychopathology (Paris, 2020b, 2022).

Throughout adult life, people continue to change, sometimes in surprising ways, often marked by turns to better functioning (Vaillant, 2012). This ubiquity of resilience carries a hopeful message: The past does not determine the present. No matter how unhappy life has been, adults have the opportunity to attain better functioning in later life.

In a clinically useful book, Southwick and Charney (2018) drew on a combination of self-report and interview data to examine what research can tell us about the key components of resilience. One of the most important is *optimism*. What we are talking about here is not foolish optimism, but an ability to recognize that life's challenges, however difficult they are, offer opportunities for psychological growth and development.

Behavioral genetics has shown that about half the variance in optimism is partially heritable (Mosing et al., 2009). But this finding, with a heritability between .34 and .46, still leaves more than half the variance to environmental factors. Moreover, there is evidence that people who are pessimistic by nature can be trained to change their view of the world (Cicchetti, 2010). That finding may have relevance for how we treat PTSD with psychotherapy.

A positive outlook on life is also linked to some of the other mechanisms proposed by Southwick and Charney (2018). These include a moral compass (a sense of what is right and wrong, and the determination to act on it) as well as faith or spirituality and a sense that life has both meaning and direction.

Another major component of resilience proposed by these authors can be best described as *facing fear*. As is well known in behavioral psychology, the best antidote to fear is "getting back on the horse." As a clinician who has specialized in personality disorders, my experience has been that avoidant personality traits are particularly difficult to manage, because fear begets even more fear and failure. Nonetheless, there is evidence that exposure is an intervention that has some role in helping people with PTSD (Foa & Meadows, 1997; Foa et al., 1989).

The final component is *social support*. We are a social species, and even the introverts among us need to have meaningful connection with a community. We also benefit from role models who have overcome adversities in life, and who inspire us to believe in our own capacities.

It is notable that all these characteristics are largely temperamental. However, while some people can more easily apply most of these strategies, that does not mean they cannot be learned. For those whose genetic inheritance makes doing so more difficult, therapists can teach skills that are better adaptations to adversity.

In summary, trauma is associated with risk but can often be overcome through resilience. Its ultimate outcome depends on temperamental characteristics and the severity of adversities.

POSTTRAUMATIC GROWTH

Finally, let us consider a concept that proposes that traumatic events can be processed in ways that lead to *posttraumatic growth* (see Tedeschi et al., 2018, for an recent summary and review of this literature). These authors have conducted research that shows that positive changes are common after trauma: appreciation of life, relationships with others, new possibilities in life, personal strength, and spiritual change. Such changes are strongly related to two of the domains described by the Five-Factor Model: Openness to Experience and Extraversion. These traits make it more possible to repair the cracked pot of trauma. Finally, research suggests that posttraumatic growth may be just as common as PTSD.

The assumption that each and every setback in life has the capacity to make people ill is not justified, and it leads to a victim-focused perspective on trauma. A good example in current affairs can be seen in the president of the United States, who became a better person after setbacks that would have paralyzed many other people.

Posttraumatic growth is the other side of survivorship and resilience. It may not happen to everyone, but it offers a more positive view of how we process life experience.

Chapter 5

Childhood Trauma and Posttraumatic Stress Disorder

CHILDHOOD TRAUMA AS A RISK FACTOR FOR PSYCHOPATHOLOGY

Early childhood trauma is an established risk factor for psychopathology (Noll, 2021). The evidence from multiple studies is clear and convincing, and the relationship has been confirmed by several meta-analyses (Amado et al., 2015; Chen et al., 2010; Dovran et al., 2015; Liu et al., 2019). However, this does not mean that every person exposed to childhood trauma will necessarily develop a mental disorder. Rather, it describes a statistical risk that affects some people, but not others.

Moreover, although childhood trauma is a risk factor for a wide range of mental disorders, posttraumatic stress disorder (PTSD) is not the most common of these outcomes. A report from the E-Risk Longitudinal Twin Study in the United Kingdom (Lewis et al., 2019) assessed a birth cohort of 2,232 twins at four time points between ages 5 and 12, with a follow-up at age 18. The results showed that 31% reported exposure to trauma but only 8% developed PTSD. The most common pathological outcomes in this cohort were major depression and conduct disorder.

These findings also apply to adolescents. In the United States, researchers conducted a large-scale epidemiological study in an urban area (Detroit) considered to be at high risk and evaluated their sample at age 21 (Breslau et al., 2004). The results were that 88% of males and 78% of females reported a past history of traumatic events, with assaultive violence most common in males and rape most common in females. Yet PTSD was diagnosed in only 6% of males and 8% of females. But this study also showed that multiple adversities greatly increase the long-term risk.

Kessler et al. (2012) reported data from a large community sample of adolescents assessed at age 13 to 17, using a supplement to the well-known National Comorbidity Survey Replication (NCS-R: Kessler et al., 1995). This project, the National Comorbidity Survey—Adolescent (NCS-A), did not directly measure the frequency of traumatic events, but about half of the subjects could be diagnosed with a mental disorder. However, only 4% of the cohort met criteria for PTSD within a 12-month frame, a much lower prevalence than the nearly 8% reported in the NCS-R.

Thus, while all these data point to a relationship between early trauma and mental disorders, the link is not reliably consistent. We must consider several caveats before jumping to conclusions.

First, the overall role of early trauma as a risk factor does not mean that it has a *specific* relationship with posttraumatic symptoms. Instead, trauma is linked to many types of adult mental disorders, of which PTSD is only one. Even when PTSD features do develop, one sees significant overlap and comorbidity with other types of symptoms and disorders.

A second issue is that most children exposed to trauma do *not* develop adult psychopathology (Fergusson et al., 1996, 1996b). This highly variable response depends on both the nature of the exposure and individual levels of resilience.

A third issue is that much of the research on childhood adversity in the community has depended on self-report, assessed years after the original event. For example, Newbury et al. (2018) did not find that self-reports and informant-report of traumatic experiences differed in their association with later psychopathology, but seemed to describe two non-overlapping populations.

A fourth issue is that traumatic events vary greatly in severity. We need to examine the *parameters* of adversities and measure the context in which they occur. As will be discussed below, this is a key issue in assessing childhood sexual abuse (CSA).

A fifth (and crucial) issue concerns what is and is not "traumatic." As we have seen, some epidemiological surveys of PTSD (e.g., Breslau et al., 1999) have been willing to see such normative events as grief or divorce as qualifying as stressors for PTSD in adults. Doing so conflates adversities that are common in life but have little else in common. Similarly, we need to focus on the most important traumas in childhood, including CSA, physical abuse, and emotional abuse, and not conflate them with the effects of dysfunctional families in the absence of clear-cut traumatic events.

A sixth issue is that adversity in adolescence needs to be considered separately from early childhood trauma. Traumatic events at that stage of development do not necessarily arise directly from parental mistreatment. While they can be seen as reflecting previous vulnerabilities and adverse experiences, many traumatic incidents in the adolescent years are perpetrated by peer groups outside the family (Fisher et al., 2015).

Finally, we need to consider whether traumatic events in childhood cause pathology in and of themselves or whether they have to be understood in a wider context of family dysfunction. The context in which trauma is most likely to become pathogenic is when children live in a dysfunctional family (Frewen et al., 2015). Children raised in such environments are more likely to be abused, both inside and outside of the family. For example, research on CSA finds that many of its effects can be accounted for by coexisting risk factors, such as a dysfunctional family environment (Fergusson & Mullen, 1999).

We also need to consider the impact of *emotional neglect*, a risk factor that often accompanies child abuse but does not really belong in a list of "traumas." Neglect is not the same as emotional abuse, in which children are harshly criticized, and it is not the same as physical neglect, in which children are not cared for. Rather, it describes a failure to understand or validate emotional reactions in children (Linehan, 1993). Emotional neglect is much more prevalent than events generally considered traumatic (Norman et al., 2012). Since child maltreatment co-occurs with parental neglect and other forms of family dysfunction, long-term risks are not always due to any specific set of experiences. Instead, psychopathology is associated with multiple adversities and with problematic childrearing as a whole (Rutter et al., 2012).

CHILDHOOD SEXUAL ABUSE

CSA carries a strong statistical risk for adult mental disorders (Fergusson & Mullen, 1999). A history of CSA is prominently (although by no means universally) reported in some adult disorders, such as borderline personality disorder (Zanarini, 2005).

Research on the long-term sequelae of CSA has been clarified by the use of meta-analyses of cross-sectional data from community populations (Rind & Tromovitch, 1997; Rind et al., 1998), as well as by prospective studies of abused children (Fergusson et al., 1996a, 1996b). Both sets of findings demonstrate that while exposure to child abuse increases the risk for developing a range of psychological symptoms, only a minority of exposed persons develop clinically significant psychopathology. (These conclusions, now widely confirmed, proved so controversial 20 years ago that Professor Rind was attacked on the floor of the U.S. Congress for publishing a scientific report—an early example of what we now call "cancel culture.")

These discrepancies between exposure and outcome are partly accounted for by differences in severity of abuse. Severity of exposure is more important than the simple presence of traumatic experiences, and it can be measured by examining the parameters of abuse, as was established several decades ago (Browne & Finkelhor, 1986). These parameters include the nature, frequency, and duration of the trauma, as well as the identity of the perpetrator. For example, there is a major difference between the impact of incest and that of extra-familial molestation. Yet above and beyond these parameters, a notable discrepancy remains between traumatic exposure and the likelihood of clinically significant sequelae (Fergusson & Mullen, 1999).

In a review of this literature, Katerndahl et al. (2005) concluded that while meta-analyses demonstrate a statistical relationship between CSA and a wide range of psychological symptoms in adulthood (including PTSD), long-term outcomes are more likely to be related to specific attributes of CSA and associated with other childhood experiences, most particularly the family environment. This finding helps explain why only a minority of those with a history of CSA develop severe psychopathology.

Nonetheless, research has shown that large numbers of children, many more than previously thought, have been exposed to CSA in some form (Finkelhor, 1990). These findings aroused great concern and point to a need to protect children from such adversities. Even if not every abused child becomes a dysfunctional adult, vulnerable children who experience these adversities are at risk for consequences. But the background for CSA is all too often emotional neglect and lack of parental supervision.

A large-scale New Zealand prospective community study (Fergusson et al., 1996a,b) was one of the few to examine the parameters of CSA in detail. It found that among incidents that involve physical contact, the perpetrator was most often a non-family member; CSA involving a blood relative accounted for only about 3% of such incidents. The most damaging scenario, father–daughter incest, is much less common than abuse from a stepfather or a mother's boyfriend or from another family member. Similarly, there is a large difference between abuse that goes on for years versus a single incident, and full intercourse is much more damaging than inappropriate touching.

In our own study of CSA in patients with BPD (Paris et al., 1994a, 1994b), we also found that examining the parameters of abuse gives a different picture of its psychopathological consequences. Thus, when we omitted single incidents that did not involve physical contact, as well as incidents involving peer groups that only occurred during adolescence, we found that no more than a third of our sample had been exposed to this kind of trauma. However, the vast majority of our patients came from dysfunctional families and described emotional neglect.

Similar considerations apply to the prevalence of CSA in the community. Finkelhor (1990) reported on a national survey in the United States in which 27% of women and 16% of men reported some form of CSA. However, half of these incidents did not involve any physical contact but consisted of either exposure to exhibitionism or simply a threatening situation. The larger numbers that have sometimes been reported are therefore misleading, and the rate of abuse that is severe enough to produce psychopathological consequences is lower. It is difficult to determine the prevalence precisely, since everything depends on what cutoff points are used. For this reason, the scary claims we sometimes hear about the ubiquity of abuse are misleading.

The good news is that in recent years, as children are being more closely supervised, rates of CSA have been falling (Finkelhor & Jones, 2006). This is the upside of "helicopter parenting." Interestingly, surveys from several countries have shown that CSA peaked in the years after the Second World War, a time when families were unusually unstable, and has been in decline for the last 30 years (Shields et al., 2016, 2019).

These conclusions should not be understood to minimize the impact of child CSA, but abuse does not happen in a vacuum. All experienced clinicians have seen cases in which CSA was a major element in the life histories of patients. What we need to keep in mind is that these effects occur in a broader environment of family dysfunction that raises the risk for its occurrence and also makes it more pathogenic.

OTHER FORMS OF CHILDHOOD MALTREATMENT

Physical abuse of children describes physical attacks that sometimes lead to significant injuries. We define physical abuse as occur in families, in which the perpetrators are caretakers. It should be kept in mind that PA in the form of spanking was until recently considered normal, but times have changed. (Of course, there is no debate about cases in which parents actually inflict injuries.) The ubiquity of physical abuse has long been a public concern, but as parenting practices change in society, the rate is also on the decline (Institute of Medicine and National Research Council, 2014). However, some children are still being beaten, and these experiences are associated with a risk for later psychopathology, although the relationship is usually weaker than for CSA (Gil, 2013; Norman et al., 2012). Again, severity has to be taken into account in making predictions about long-term outcome. Finally, physical abuse, like CSA, usually occurs in a climate of family dysfunction (Gil, 2013).

Emotional abuse is a form of maltreatment in which caretakers are harshly and consistently critical of children in words and actions (Loring, 1994). Even if there is no physical contact, emotional abuse can be mentally damaging. This form of mistreatment has been the subject of a large amount of research and even has its own journal. Emotional abuse is more frequently reported by patients than CSA or physical abuse, and it has effects as significant as other forms of maltreatment. Its impact might be understood in terms of reducing self-esteem in children. But unlike CSA and physical abuse, the frequency of emotional abuse has not been shown to have diminished over recent decades (Institute of Medicine and National Research Council, 2014).

EMOTIONAL NEGLECT

Emotional neglect describes a failure of caretakers to understand and acknowledge the feelings of children. While it qualifies as the most common form of maltreatment (Institute of Medicine and National Research Council, 2014), emotional neglect should not be considered a form of trauma. That is because it is not an episode but rather a pattern of interaction that stretches over the entire period of childhood development. Although the concept of neglect is crucial for understanding risk factors for mental disorders, this adversity has often been neglected in research (Boyce & Malhomes, 2013). A longitudinal study found that emotional neglect during childhood has a significant association with depression and substance use in young adults (Cohen et al., 2017).

Emotional neglect is associated with a theoretical principle: Children have powerful emotions that they have difficulty controlling and regulating, and there is considerable variation in the intensity of these feelings (Gross, 2014). These problems can be prominent in childhood but tend to become less intense as the brain matures, leading to better control of the limbic system by the frontal cortex. But families also play an important role in the learning process. When children are upset, they need a caretaker to soothe them and calm them down. Some parents are better at this than others. When children's emotions are dismissed and invalidated, they can build up to a toxic level, as in the emotion dysregulation that so frequently characterizes patients who suffer from BPD (Linehan, 1993).

Yet like abuse, emotional neglect cannot be understood in isolation. Research again shows that pathways to mental disorders tend to be governed by the continuous and cumulative effects of a dysfunctional family environment (Cicchetti, 2005; Rutter et al., 2012). Thus, emotional neglect is another childhood adversity that is most likely to happen when parenting is emotionally insensitive and/or chaotic.

Research also demonstrates the effects of extreme neglect early in development. The best and most thoroughly researched example is the outcome for Romanian orphans who had been placed in cribs at birth, left there for months on end, and given almost no care except for feeding. While I have cast doubt on the idea that early adversity is always pathogenic, when neglect is that severe, it interferes with brain development. The brain matures rapidly in the first few years of life, and this process strongly depends on environmental input.

Some of these children from Romania were adopted by families in the United Kingdom and the United States, allowing for what Rutter et al. (2004) called a "natural experiment", in which a highly neglectful environment was replaced by a much better one. The longer these children had spent in the orphanage, the more difficult it was for them to develop normally later in life. While many of the deficits remained subtle and did not severely affect adult functioning, those most severely affected had measurable neuropsychological deficits and problems relating properly to other people. This research shows that when it is this extreme, early emotional deprivation can cause lasting damage. Yet at the same time, the majority of these orphans eventually developed normally by their young adult years. Thus, the findings of these studies also demonstrate the importance of resilience.

ATTACHMENT, TEMPERAMENT, AND TRAUMA

Childhood trauma cannot be understood without considering the larger role of a psychological and social environment. It also cannot be understood without considering temperamental differences between children.

One of the most influential models of child development is *attachment theory*. This theoretical structure offers a useful context for understanding both trauma and neglect. Originally developed by the British psychoanalyst John Bowlby (1969), it has been the subject of a large body of research (Cassidy & Shaver, 2016). Simply put, attachment theory focuses on the needs of children for protection and emotional security, and it hypothesizes that an absence of secure attachments in early life is a major risk factor for mental disorders in later life.

Children who grow up in dysfunctional families marked by parental psychopathology and high levels of conflict, along with abuse and neglect, are also likely to suffer from failures in attachment. Again, since resilience is common, these relationships are statistical and not fully predictable. Also, the effects of attachment failures can be subtle, sometimes apparent in adult interpersonal relationships as a lack of trust.

Variations in temperament are crucial for understanding the long-term impact of childhood trauma. This is because temperament and personality have a major heritable component, as shown in behavioral genetic research (Knopik et al., 2017). This same principle can even be observed in general medicine: Immune responses to infections, such as COVID-19, are more concordant in monozygotic than in dizygotic twins (Williams et al., 2020).

Surprisingly, there has long been intense hostility in mainstream psychology to even talking about heritability (Plomin, 2018). Many are afraid of the conclusion that genetics is destiny. Others are afraid of having their expertise absorbed by another discipline. Still others believe that psychology can make the world better and would rather not think about genes. Resistance among psychotherapists to considering the role of heritability is based on the mistaken idea that genes are deterministic. Actually, while genes bend the twig, they do not predict the final form of the tree. Instead of either genetic determinism or psychosocial determinism, we need to adopt a point of view in which the effects of the psychosocial environment are understood as interacting with heritable traits.

Temperament helps to explain why the outcome of trauma can be so variable. While a predisposed and vulnerable minority will be badly affected by early experiences, many people who have had an unhappy childhood function reasonably well as adults (Rutter et al., 2012). Again, the effects of trauma are also most likely to persist when stressors are multiple, when they are repeated, and when they fail to be counteracted by positive experiences (Rutter & Rutter, 1993). In short, while resilience is ubiquitous, even the strongest constitution can be brought down by a severe and continued onslaught.

One of the most important lines of research has examined the *interactions* between childhood trauma and temperament. The best known is the research of Caspi et al. (2002, 2003), which found that effects of traumatic experiences early in life are more likely to produce symptoms in those who have specific alleles affecting serotonin (associated with depression) or monoamine oxidase activity (associated with antisocial behavior). These findings support an interactive model, but they have remained controversial, as other studies have failed to replicate them (Fergusson et al., 2011). The main problem is that it is unlikely that outcomes as complex as mental disorders can be accounted for by single genes. Psychopathological outcomes are most likely to emerge due to interactions between many genes and many life events.

In other words, we need to invoke a biopsychosocial model of psychopathology (Engel, 1980). In addition to heritable temperament and life experiences, social risk factors also play a role in the vulnerability to PTSD and to other mental disorders (Auxéméry, 2012). This relationship is also notable for substance abuse and eating disorders (Paris, 2020d).

I am skeptical about the idea that social factors in modern life have promoted child abuse. We often hear the claim that the problems of modern society are getting worse, that people are more unhappy, and that "the good old days" were better. Yet the social climate of the past was not good for most of us. By almost any measure, the present is the best time to live in human history (Pinker, 2019). The evidence clearly shows that abuse is much less common than it once was. In the past, physical maltreatment of children was ubiquitous and was considered perfectly normal and even necessary. Yet recent decades have shown a marked decrease in early trauma of all kinds, including sexual and physical abuse. If anything, today's families may have moved too far in the direction of overprotection (Lukianoff & Haidt, 2018). Moreover, even as parenting practices have become more benign, the overall prevalence of mental disorders has not changed over recent decades (Patten et al., 2006). Those diagnoses that seem to have gone up with time are more likely to reflect changes in diagnostic practice than in society.

In summary, the relationship between early trauma and adult functioning involves highly complex pathways. Understanding them can help treatment if patients are encouraged to replace blaming others for psychological problems by moving on and developing feelings of agency and empowerment in their adult lives.

ARE EARLIER EXPERIENCES MORE IMPORTANT THAN LATER EXPERIENCES?

The primacy of childhood risk factors over later life events tends to be taken as an axiom. But why *should* early events be more important? Several possible answers have been proposed. Here I will follow the work of Jerome Kagan (1998), who has provided a useful and detailed critique of these assumptions.

The first issue is that early learning occurs when the brain is more plastic. Thus, infants, who have not previously been exposed to a social environment, might be more profoundly or permanently affected by the quality of parenting. The second is that early learning occurs during sensitive periods of development, when the organism is primed to learn certain patterns more easily. A third is that early learning occurs when the child is more dependent, making younger children most susceptible to the influence of parents.

The first argument, concerning plasticity, fails to take into account that even if infants are born without prior experience, each child begins life with unique temperamental characteristics. Moreover, individual differences in temperament are a major determinant of parental responses (Harris, 1998). There is also little evidence that emotional responses in children are more plastic in infancy than later on in development. Events in the early years might even be *less* important, since most memories of this period are lost, and few can remember life events before age 3. Very early events might affect children on a nonverbal level, but infants and toddlers lack the cognitive maturity to evaluate their experience. The brain is still growing in the first 2 years of life, and the frontal lobes, where experience is evaluated, are particularly immature.

The second argument, concerning sensitive periods of development, is also open to serious question. Kagan (1998), reviewing the literature on imprinting of animals in the wild, and on early separation from maternal care in laboratory animals, concludes that sensitive periods are much less important in human children, who are born with a more flexible program for learning. (Yet, as discussed earlier, unusually severe neglect can interfere with these developmental pathways.) Kagan was also critical of some popular ideas of the late 20th century, such as that mothers must provide increased stimulation to help infants lay down neural networks, that bonding must begin through physical contact in the first few hours of life, or that children benefit from prenatal exposure to music.

Kagan (1998, pp. 126–127) usefully describes how emotional reactions to traumatic events early in childhood can become dulled over time:

Most adults experience the gradual loss, over time, of strong emotional reactions, perhaps fear of an animal, sadness over the death of a parent, anger at a rival, or intense sexual arousal at the sight or thought of another. It strains credulity to argue that infants are exceptions to this universal aspect of human nature and do not lose emotional reactions acquired during the first two years of life.

The third argument, concerning the dependency of young children, is correct up to a point, but research shows that in many if not most cases, a later more positive environment can modify the influence of early rearing. While risk can be raised by early adversity, there need be no *consistent* or *permanent* effects from leaving infants alone and untended for long periods, from being separated from a mother, from being in day care, or even from experiencing multiple fostering or life in an orphanage (Kagan, 1998).

Moreover, if childrearing practices during infancy and early childhood were as important as is often claimed, we should see dramatic differences in the frequency of psychological problems that accord with cultural variations. Yet the prevalence of serious mental disorders is about the same around the world.

In summary, there is no definitive evidence that adversity necessarily has a greater effect earlier in life than it does later. Adversities that begin early usually tend to continue over time, creating the *illusion* that timing is a crucial factor. It is possible that early adversity can create feedback loops that make it more difficult for improvements in the environment to take effect. But resilience, the natural state of most children, is a mechanism that can only be overridden by continued environmental stress. Thus, the persistence of adversity over time is much more important than what happens at any particular stage of development.

Once again, to quote Kagan (1998, pp. 128–129):

> Those who favor infant determinism do not award sufficient power to the events of later childhood and adolescence, many of which are correlated with social class. One of the few robust facts in the social sciences is that a person's social class predicts the probability of school failure, violent crime, choice of vocation, and physical and mental symptoms . . . If an adult has impairing symptoms, it is more reasonable to attribute them to the continuous influence of an adverse environment than to conclude that the symptoms represent the untouched traces of early neglect.

The course of life is never fully determined. By and large, discontinuities are the rule in development. There can always be changes, some for the better, others for the worse. These facts led one well-known developmental psychologist (Lewis, 1997) to publish a book-length critique of the primacy of early experience. Suspicious of determinism, this author offered the optimistic view that it is always possible to alter one's fate, and that one does not necessarily need therapy to accomplish this goal. Moreover, Lewis, drawing on a wide literature in social psychology, argued that behavior is highly contextual and emphasized that people behave very differently in different environments. Rutter (2013) summarized a series of observations about "turning points" in development. Meeting new people, moving to a new neighborhood, or attending a new school can break cycles of disadvantage.

Thus, the primacy of early adversity may be largely accounted for by children whose temperamental vulnerability prevents them from taking advantage of their environment, leading to a vicious cycle between genes and environment. But the good news is that given a change in their luck, most adults with a traumatic childhood can go on to lead productive lives.

Chapter 6

Trauma and the Science of Memory

Modern psychotherapy is well over a century old, and the professions that provide psychological treatments have matured. Therapists today use more sophisticated theoretical models and rely more on evidence-based interventions. Nonetheless, some clinicians still hold a belief that childhood trauma is not only a major risk factor for psychopathology but that it also tends not to be remembered. This chapter will show that this point of view is contradicted by research into the science of memory. Needless to say, memories that are false cannot account for posttraumatic stress disorder (PTSD).

THE RECOVERED MEMORY MOVEMENT

The modern recovered memory movement took off after the publication of an influential book on childhood trauma by Judith Herman (1992). Herman laid down the gauntlet (on p. 5) by stating that "the ordinary response to atrocities is to banish them from consciousness." This radical claim was made without any support from empirical evidence.

However, Herman's concept of "complex PTSD," a disorder deriving from multiple traumatic events that affect personality development, has gained more traction. (It will be discussed in Chapter 7.) But the idea that traumatic episodes are "usually" repressed runs contrary to one of the key features of PTSD: the presence of intrusive traumatic memories. If Herman's model were correct, it would run up against the way painful memories return to consciousness no matter how hard people try to forget them. PTSD is not characterized by amnesia but rather by "hypermnesia" (excessive memory), which is one of the principal criteria for the disorder in the fifth edition of the *Diagnostic and Statistical Manual of Mental Disorders* (American Psychiatric Association, 2013).

Herman proposed that even when patients did not remember having been subjected to child abuse, if they have symptoms that could be accounted for by such experiences, memories for these events must have been repressed. Therefore, one of the aims of therapy would be to recover and process these memories. This may be the most dangerous aspect of her views. It harks back to Sigmund Freud, who insisted that his patients had repressed memories and who used his authority to convince them that this was the case. (He later changed his mind.)

In the 1990s, the concept of repressed and recovered memories of abuse was further popularized in a book, *The Courage to Heal*, written by two teachers with no mental health training; it went on to sell a million copies (Bass & Davis, 1994). These authors proposed that in people with all sorts of psychological symptoms, not remembering trauma is actually a *proof* that memories have been repressed. This view was in accord with Herman's idea that forgetting is a usual response to trauma. But its assumption that data that run contrary to theory actually prove the opposite is a typical feature of conspiracy theories.

One of the early ideas of Freud (1896) was the assumption that all life events are fully recorded in the brain as memories, even if they are not readily accessible. We now know that this is not true: The brain is a bit like a computer in that it has limited storage and is not a repository for all life events. We *need* to forget most of the events that happen to us, and problems arise when we cannot do so. Moreover, our memories change with time, and tend to be revised each time we access them (Schacter, 2008).

Therapists influenced by these beliefs will search for repressed childhood traumas in their patients, even when memories for such events are not present. The idea that trauma is too painful to be remembered derives from Freud's view of the unconscious mind. In that theory, memories of traumatic events are like hidden abscesses, boring at the psyche from within and creating symptoms.

Paradoxically, this return to Freud coincided with a period of disillusionment with psychoanalysis in mainstream psychiatry and clinical psychology (Paris, 2012, 2019). However, Freud's psycho-analytic model has been radically revised over time, coming to focus less on real life events and more on intrapsychic conflict. In the view of those who believe in the concept of recovered memories, analytic theory took a wrong turn by downgrading fantasy in favor of reality. Giving back a central importance to traumatic events and repression was seen a welcome revival of older but still fertile ideas.

Crucially, the view that traumatic memories tend to be repressed is not consistent with the science of memory. Consider, for example, studies of Holocaust survivors (Eaton et al., 1982) and of veterans who endured life-threatening combat (Dohrenwend et al., 2006). Neither of these groups has ever been described as having forgotten what happened to them. (However, survivors may not talk about painful memories.)

Nor is there any serious evidence that abused children repress memories of traumatic events (McNally, 2003). There is a rather small literature on PTSD in children (Scheeringa, 2008), but what we know does not support the idea that impaired memory is common. Again, those who survive may be, understandably, reluctant to talk about painful events. At all ages, people tend to protect themselves by putting them out of mind or by not seeing them as traumatic. But that does not mean they do not remember what happened.

The recovered memory movement was a fad that emerged, surged, and then declined (McHugh, 2008). It seems fair to say that the skeptics have prevailed. The problem was that memories that are "uncovered" in therapy are almost certain to be factually untrue, as no evidence shows that they can be independently confirmed. Such phenomena can therefore be called *false memories*.

Thus the belief that patients suffer from repressed childhood trauma has receded in recent years but has not disappeared (Otgaar et al., 2020). In a best-selling book, van der Kolk (2014) argued that the effects of early trauma can be seen in the body, which "keeps the score." The continued popularity of these ideas (van der Kolk has been at the top of the list of paperbacks for years) is in line with theories based on a narrative of victimhood and survival that remains seductively appealing.

While it lasted, the recovered memory fad did real damage. Families were shattered by false accusations of sexual abuse. For example, a survey by Otgaar et al. (2020) documented family estrangement as one of the consequences of this kind of therapy. In addition, some day care workers were sent to jail by juries who had been instructed by prosecutors to "believe the children." Adult patients in therapy were convinced that they must have been sexually abused as children on the basis of symptoms that are in no way specific to any life event (Loftus & Ketcham, 1994). Moreover, by misidentifying abuse that had never happened, a serious disservice was also done to those who had truly been victimized. All in all, some of the harm associated with the recovered memory fad was permanent.

The general public holds a number of misconceptions about memory (Lynn et al., 2015). Many think of it as a kind of video recorder where everything that happens to people can be stored. A recent survey also found that the idea of repression after trauma is commonly believed by clinical psychologists (Ost et al., 2017). Having lived through the peak of the recovered memory fad in the 1990s, I had the impression that most clinicians remained skeptical but preferred to avoid confrontations with true believers, who were quite aggressive in their promotion of these ideas. Only a few academics, such as Paul McHugh of Johns Hopkins University, took a strong and courageous public stand against the tide (McHugh memorably made his case in 1997 on the TV program "60 Minutes").

SUPPRESSION, REPRESSION, AND DISSOCIATION

We do not remember most of what happens to us in our lives. (This is probably fortunate.) Moreover, there is a difference between *suppression* of painful memories (not thinking about them) and *repression*, which purportedly moves recollections of traumatic events to the unconscious mind, where they cannot be accessed. There is little doubt that we all have an unconscious mind. But is that a Freudian unconscious, in which access to our hidden desires is blocked, or a cognitive unconscious (Kihlstrom, 1987), in which many mental activities work automatically? Similarly, we all make use of defense mechanisms, and people are rather good at fooling themselves (Nesse, 2019). But that does not mean that memories of trauma can be locked away by repression.

A century after Freud, we lack convincing proof that the phenomenon of repressed memory exists. Decades ago, Holmes (1990, pp. 98–99) summarized the research literature on repression as follows:

> One cannot prove the null hypothesis, and therefore we cannot conclude that repression does not exist, but after sixty years of research has failed to reveal evidence for repression, it seems reasonable to question whether continued expenditure of effort on this topic is justified. Regardless of how fascinating the repression hypothesis is, the time may have come to move on.

No research finding emerged in the following decades to challenge this conclusion (McNally, 2006; Otgaar et al., 2021; Piper et al., 2008). Nor is this idea supported by clinical observations of traumatic exposure. For example, in a famous study of a kidnapping on a school bus (Terr, 1988), children who had been frightened by the experience tried to suppress the event but, like adults with PTSD, continued to be troubled by memories and found it difficult to stop thinking about what had happened to them. Moreover, most of them got the facts wrong, embroidering their memories with a multitude of false details.

In the famous phrase of 19th-century evolutionist Thomas Huxley, even the most beautiful theory can be slain by one ugly fact. But ideas that have a taste of drama, and purport to solve mysteries, are attractive and difficult to give up. We see much the same mechanism today in politics, where conspiracy theories have a way of running riot and, once promoted through the media, are difficult to remove from the public discourse.

Dissociation is another mechanism that has been invoked to explain why traumatic memories may not be accessible. A contemporary of Freud, Pierre Janet (1907), introduced this construct (the original French term was *désagrégation*). This construct describes a more radical form of forgetting in which entire segments of the mind and memory are cut off from consciousness. Dissociation has been invoked to account for certain dramatic clinical phenomena (e.g., amnesia and multiple personality). These phenomena were first described during Janet's time, but until the epidemic of "dissociative disorders" in the 1980s and 1990s, most clinicians considered these symptoms to be rare. These conditions seem to be so rare that it is doubtful that they have ever existed, except in the world of fantasy, promoted by certain forms of therapy.

Like repression, the construct of dissociation cannot readily be measured in an accurate or reliable way. Dissociation is also rather heterogeneous and includes phenomena that are not specific to trauma, such as depersonalization or derealization. Both are common in panic attacks, and many people depersonalize in the face of extreme stressors. The problem of assessing these phenomena has not been solved by the use of self-report measures, such as the Dissociative Experiences Scale (DES; Bernstein & Putnam, 1986). As there is no gold standard for comparison, these instruments have only been validated by concordance with clinical observation—which is to say they may not be valid at all.

It is well documented that dissociative symptoms are common in PTSD, and in DSM-5, dissociation is now highlighted as defining a subtype. But these phenomena are not specific to trauma, nor do they necessarily involve loss of memory, not to speak of "dissociative disorders." In a large community sample, Mulder et al. (1998) found that dissociative symptoms are common in the population but are either weakly related or unrelated to histories of childhood abuse.

My research group was interested in the relationship of these phenomena to borderline personality disorder (BPD). We found that BPD patients had unusually high levels of dissociative symptoms but that scores on the DES were related more closely to the BPD diagnosis than to specific childhood experiences (Zweig-Frank et al., 1994). In a second study (Jang et al., 1998), we gave the DES to a twin sample and documented that scores had a heritability of 45%, a typical finding for clinical phenomena of all kinds. These results suggest that a capacity to dissociate is related to underlying personality traits governing a tendency to fantasize.

Unfortunately, the concept of dissociation became central to the description of "dissociative disorders," purported to have been caused by childhood trauma (Paris, 2012). A few very rare cases fitting this description have been described over the last 100 years. However, later research suggests that memories of trauma in these patients only appear under strong suggestion from therapists (McHugh, 2008). Since patients tend to work hard to please their therapists (and may wish to be unusual and fascinating), they may be willing to develop these "alter" personalities once they are in therapy. It is doubtful as to whether anyone with these experiences has had them prior to seeing a therapist or reading about them. They remained rare for many decades, even after the publication of a best-selling book (later a movie), *The Three Faces of Eve* (Thigpen & Cleckley, 1957), which claimed to describe such a case.

The effects on public opinion were much greater for another best-seller (Schreiber, 1973), describing the most famous of these patients, Shirley Mason, who was called "Sibyl" by the author. (I remember this book being serialized in my daily newspaper at the time, and how it made me wonder why my professional life was so dull.) In the end the entire story of Sibyl turned out to be a fraud (Nathan, 2011). Mason was shown to have had a normal childhood. It was also established that she had agreed to play along with the idea of recovered memories and multiple personalities to please her therapist, Cornelia Wilbur. (When seeing a substitute psychiatrist, Mason had no reason to play the role, and once she established that the therapist was not that interested, she moved to other subjects.) Moreover, Mason and Wilbur developed a close relationship, even taking holidays together. Another serious breach of therapeutic norms was that both benefited financially from the publication of Schreiber's book (Nathan, 2011).

Unfortunately, dissociative disorders, including dissociative identity disorder (DID, equivalent to multiple personality disorder), were accepted into DSM-III. They are still to be found, in much the same form, in DSM-5. Much of the credit (if one can call it that) belongs to the Stanford University psychiatrist David Spiegel, who has chaired committees on this group of diagnoses for several editions of the DSM. The concept seems to die hard. Some articles in the media have quoted Spiegel's claim (with no reference to contrary points of view) that DID affects 1% of the population.

Unfortunately, the continued presence of DID in the DSM provides unjustified validation for true believers in these phenomena. Clinicians who make this diagnosis find themselves in a hall of mirrors in which dissociated personalities ("alters") come and go, each with its own story to tell. Obviously, there is something appealing about the bizarre and the fantastic. Yet in the end, dissociative disorders are only diagnosed by members of the cult that supports it, and they are almost never seen in clinical practice or outpatient clinics (Paris, 2012). Unlike other mental disorders, they only appear in people who are in therapy with clinicians who believe in the concept and press patients to give them the material to support that view. But the presence of dissociative disorders in a standard diagnostic manual means that every textbook has to have a chapter on them. The best one can hope for is that these clinical symptoms, and the mistaken ideas behind them, will disappear once their advocates pass from the scene.

In the end, research contradicts the ideas behind "recovered memories" in any form. The most likely explanation for the impact of these theories is the power of suggestion, the appeal of narrative, and a cultural context in which so many parents worry about what can happen to children if they fall into the wrong hands.

WHAT SCIENCE TELLS US ABOUT MEMORY

Over the last few decades, research on how memory works has shown that memories are *not* retained as accurate records of past events. Instead, all memories are *reconstructions* that are greatly modified by recent experiences (Schacter, 2008).

We do not remember most of the events that happen to us in our lives. Even when memories are emotionally significant, what we retain are narratives "rewritten" after the fact. In short, as a very large body of research has shown (Lynn et al., 2015) most people, even though their memories of past events in their own lives are unreliable, have unscientific ideas about the accuracy of memory. Moreover, the fact that very little remains in memory from the first few years of human life is not due to repression but rather to the immaturity of the brain (McNally, 2003). Even the most notable or shocking events in our lives, which were once thought to create "flashbulb memories," only yield edited versions of the past. Later recall does not match records of events that were written down at the time of a potentially traumatic incident; instead, memories are revised in the light of later events (Schacter, 2001, 2008). Thus, the supposedly photographic recall of dramatic events is a myth, and memories become more and more distorted over time (McNally, 2003).

The fact that people do not remember events precisely has been known for some time: The first major study of the inaccuracy of memory was published nine decades ago (Bartlett, 1932). The findings showed that the farther in the past the original event was, the more likely it is that a memory will be distorted.

Actually, it would not make sense if memory represented a detailed record of every event in our lives. The brain is faced with constant environmental input, so that what is recorded for future reference requires serious screening. In spite of the enormous storage capacity of the brain, recording *all* input would be highly inefficient. Like the hard disk on the computer or an overstuffed filing cabinet, the mind can become overloaded with information it does not need.

Memory systems must therefore be selective. There is no need to keep precise records of every detail of our lives. For this reason, memories are overall impressions that are rarely factually accurate and that include many elements of imaginative reconstruction. What is recorded is *processed*, so that preexisting cognitive schemata influence the ultimate record of events. And each time we retrieve a memory, it is edited in the light of subsequent events. Memories are, therefore, *interactions* between actual events and preconceived ideas (Loftus & Ketcham, 1994).

Moreover, memory is a very complex system, with separate mechanisms for remembering a name, a behavioral sequence, everyday life events, or childhood events (Schacter, 2008). There is also an important distinction between *explicit* memories (involving the encoding of actual experiences) and *implicit* memories (involving the encoding of skills). These subsystems make use of different neurophysiological pathways. Implicit memories are generally unconscious, but that does not mean that they correspond to the unconscious mind proposed by Freud (Kihlstrom, 1987).

Another idea that has had a fair amount of currency with certain clinicians (and with the public at large) is that traumatic events, when repressed, produce a strong "imprint" on the mind and body. Thus, even when the mind denies the truth, it has been claimed that the body remembers and "keeps the score" (van der Kolk, 2014). One piece of information that is most often quoted in favor of this idea is that trauma can change activity in the hypothalamic–pituitary–adrenal axis; another is that patients with PTSD often have a smaller hippocampus (Yehuda, 2002). But we do not know whether such findings reflect the effects of trauma, represent a broader comorbid pattern, or serve as markers for a biological vulnerability to trauma that can be observed prior to the development of symptoms.

Moreover, events associated with strong emotion are not remembered more accurately than those of less significance. As documented in many experiments, eyewitness testimony is surprisingly inaccurate, because memories reflect as much of what people expect to see as what they actually see (Loftus & Ketcham, 1994). As already noted, these findings have had an important influence on the legal system, which is now less likely to be automatically reliant on eyewitnesses.

Thus, no objective method, short of corroborating data, can determine whether any memory is true or false. And it is surprisingly easy to create false memories that are reported with enormous conviction (Loftus & Ketcham, 1994). Individuals can then add telling details that seem to support the veracity of the story, at least to a naive observer.

The use of hypnosis as a means of recovering memories only makes recall less accurate (Lynn et al., 2015). In fact, memories obtained by hypnosis are much more likely to be false. Under hypnosis, one can implant highly detailed, but untrue, memories of past events. While such studies do not involve real traumatic events, the mechanisms of memory formation are not different.

LESSONS FROM THE RECOVERED MEMORY EPIDEMIC

The epidemic of recovered memories, in which patients seem to remember traumatic events after years of forgetting, was the product of fantasy and/or therapist suggestions. Children are generally more suggestible than adults, as one can see in a series of court cases in which children were aggressively pushed by interviews into supporting accusations of abuse against day care workers (McHugh, 2008). This led to innocent people being sent to prison, and, for a time, working in a day care center became a hazardous occupation.

Moreover, searching for recovered memories in clinical situations can have a negative impact on patients. When accusations turn out to be false, the ensuing shattering of families is a major side effect. Future observers may see this scandal as a folly inviting ridicule, but it is patients and their families who have had to bear the brunt of incorrect theories.

Yet for several decades, the recovered memory controversy polarized psychotherapists. Because of the intensity of the controversy, some still prefer to believe that reality must lie between two extremes. Brewin and Andrews (1998) defended an approach that allows for the existence of recovered memories, claiming that their point of view is "balanced." But research is not like television, where crackpots often get an audience when the goal is to be "fair and balanced" between opposing views.

Science is a hard taskmaster that requires us to question our most cherished beliefs. We may want to look at both sides of a controversy, but sometimes the answer is that one side is dead wrong. In the end, belief in repression and recovered memories is an example of pseudoscience. It is bad to be balanced when psychological theories and methods are not only wrong but also dangerous.

The recovered memory "movement" will probably go down in the history of clinical psychology and psychiatry as one of their greatest scandals, creating a cult that sometimes threatened to bring the practice of psychotherapy itself into disrepute. One of the most troubling aspects of this controversy has been that those who disagree with the validity of recovered memories can be attacked as being somehow against feminism. But one cannot sacrifice science in the service of ideology.

Trauma remains a highly emotional issue. We live in a society that is deeply concerned about the protection of children, and about harm inflicted on the innocent. The worldwide scandal about child abuse in the Catholic Church is a prominent example. But we also live in a society where, in most families, both parents need to work, leaving their children in the care of others for extended periods. Doing so has been crucial in bringing women into the workforce. These tensions may help explain why false accusations of child abuse became more common about 30 years ago.

Ironically, we now know much more about child maltreatment, and we better understand its relationship to long-term sequelae. This research teaches us to think about risks in a more nuanced way. It is a mistake to put all forms of childhood trauma into the same box. It is also a mistake to fail to consider the dysfunctional contexts in which traumatic events occur. Another pitfall for clinicians is that patients may present them with the kind of material that supports their theories. If they probe aggressively for traumatic memories, and show more interest when they are produced, further elaboration to the point of confabulation may follow. In contrast, even if past events are acknowledged and discussed, the main emphasis should be on dysfunction in a patient's current life. In short, there is no magic to treatment that focuses on traumatic memories. Patients tend to get better when they put their past behind them and have the courage to build a better life.

The main lesson of the recovered memory movement is that mental health clinicians need to guard against simplistic ideas that belong in a movie script. The effects of trauma can be powerful, but they are impossible to predict. Mental health clinicians must learn to work with complexity and unpredictability.

Chapter 7

Posttraumatic Stress Disorder, Personality Disorders, and Complex Posttraumatic Stress Disorder

POSTTRAUMATIC STRESS DISORDER IN THE CONTEXT OF PERSONALITY

Since 1980, with the introduction of the system outlined in the third edition of the *Diagnostic and Statistical Manual of Mental Disorders* (DSM-III; American Psychiatric Association, 1980), clinicians have become accustomed to make diagnoses that require patients to meet a given number of criteria listed in a manual. In most cases, if more than half of the criteria are present, one can make a diagnosis. But psychopathology is more than a collection of symptoms that need to be counted. This rather mechanical (and not very evidence-based) procedure fails to consider that psychological symptoms reflect the functioning of underlying mental structures. These can be assessed by the wider domains of psychopathology, such as externalizing and internalizing disorders (Kotov et al., 2017), as well as personality trait profiles and personality disorders (Costa & Widiger, 2015).

Clinicians focus on symptoms because they want to target them with specific methods of treatment. But it is often more useful to view them in a matrix in which biological, psychological, and social vulnerabilities interact within a complex network. This approach can be used to develop a statistical procedure called *network analysis*, which examines patterns of relationships between risk factors and life events within a model describing interactions that have a causal structure (Hevey, 2018). Several researchers have applied network analysis to understanding the etiology of posttraumatic stress disorder (PTSD; Armour et al., 2017; McNally et al., 2017). The idea behind this procedure is to account for less-than-predictable outcomes by describing points of strong interaction between risks and symptoms can be identified. Some researchers think it has the potential to offer a new approach to understanding psychopathology (Borsboom & Cramer, 2013). However, network analysis is not totally different from the DSM, in that it depends entirely on clinical symptoms and does not offer an etiological explanation for mental disorders.

In PTSD, physiological reactivity in response to reminders of the trauma drives many of its clinical symptoms (McNally et al., 2017). As we have seen, high levels of reactivity to the environment are a key feature of Neuroticism. The tendency to develop depression or anxiety is rooted in this trait, which governs the intensity and duration of responses to environmental challenges (Everly & Lating, 2019). These relationships are most understandable in the context of personality trait profiles.

Clinicians who are impressed by posttraumatic symptoms may not always see PTSD within the framework of personality. Yet we cannot understand responses to stressors without taking these trait profiles into account. It is personality that determines how strongly people react to stressors, as we have seen in relation to Neuroticism and PTSD. In a larger context, it makes sense to conclude that psychological symptoms of all kinds emerge from a matrix of underlying traits.

Personality is therefore a *psychological immune system* that determines how experiences are processed. Like the physical immune system, these reactions can be protective against symptoms, but they can also lead to complications if associated with an overactive response to stressors.

PERSONALITY TRAITS AND PSYCHOLOGICAL SYMPTOMS

Personality describes features of thought, emotion, and behavior that vary between individuals. Understanding inborn temperamental variations, and the personality trait profiles that they shape, requires an evolutionary perspective (Beck et al., 2015; Nesse, 2019). Personality shows individual variation because trait profiles are a kind of evolutionary hedge, in that traits can be adaptive or maladaptive in different environments. Thus, Neuroticism will be adaptive in an environment that is unpredictably dangerous, but it can be maladaptive when the brain's alarm system cannot be turned off. At that point, traits begin to interfere with functioning, and symptoms of anxiety, depression, or PTSD can be framed within a broader diagnosis—that is, personality disorder.

The broad dimensions of the Five-Factor Model of personality (Costa & Widiger, 2015) are the most widely used framework for describing trait profiles. They describe five domains, which can be remembered using the acronym "OCEAN" (Openness to Experience, Conscientiousness, Extraversion, Agreeableness, and Neuroticism). Openness (related to creativity) and Extraversion (related to the need to be with people) do not have strong clinical implications. But extremes on the other three dimensions (Neuroticism, Conscientiousness, and Agreeableness) are associated with a vulnerability to psychopathology. Most of the patients clinicians see, particularly those presenting with anxiety and depression, are high in Neuroticism. Patients with personality disorders usually have this trait, but they are also low in Conscientiousness and Agreeableness. In other words, these patients are not just afraid or sad but also have dysfunctional interpersonal relationships and problems in the workplace.

We see patients who are overly conscientious, a feature of personality that, if extreme, can also interfere with functioning in both work and intimate relationships. On the other hand, being too low in Conscientiousness is associated with impulsivity and severe personality dysfunction. There are times when reacting more impulsively can be adaptive (as in rapid responses to situations of danger). And those who are overly conscientious are hard to live with or work with.

We also see patients who are highly disagreeable, which also affects work and intimacy. But some patients get into trouble by being overly agreeable, allowing other people to take advantage of that trait. Each of these extremes can be the right reaction under some conditions and the wrong reaction under others.

Neuroticism is most strongly related to a vulnerability to PTSD. Being low on this trait can be adaptive if one is not facing significant life stressors but maladaptive if one's emotions are too readily dismissed. People vulnerable to PTSD have overly strong reactions to all kinds of potential and actual adverse events, and these reactions often lead to dysfunction in work and relationships—that is, to personality disorder.

Let us return to the analogy with the body's immune system. It is essential to have immune responses to microbial parasites, but an overly sensitive system may turn on normal body cells and lead to autoimmune diseases. It is now well established that early exposure to viruses (such as polio) prevents more severe disease later in development. Moreover, while some foods (such as peanuts) can stimulate problematic responses of the immune system in some people, an overly thorough protection against exposure to stressors early in life can lead to dangerous overreactions later on.

Given these striking individual differences in vulnerability, we need not assume that susceptibility to psychological trauma is universal, or that everyone is intrinsically fragile. Some social scientists have proposed that contemporary society views young people in just this way, instead of encouraging them to learn from experience and become "anti-fragile" (Taleb, 2012). Prominent social psychologists have criticized contemporary parenting as overprotective, denying young people the opportunity to become stronger by mastering adversity (Lukianoff & Haidt, 2018; Twenge et al., 2019). Campbell and Manning (2018) argue that defining oneself as a victim has replaced older values based on honor and shame, and that suffering has almost become a source of prestige in modern society. This point of view also affects psychotherapists, who may be tempted to allow patients to blame their families (or society as a whole) for their problems, rather than taking on agency and ownership over their life.

CHILDHOOD TRAUMA, PTSD, AND BORDERLINE PERSONALITY DISORDER

There is a very large body of research on borderline personality disorder (BPD; Paris, 2020a). Patients who suffer from this condition suffer from marked mood instability, unstable intimate relationships, and a wide range of impulsive behaviors (particularly self-harm and suicide attempts). Linehan (1993) hypothesized that emotional dysregulation (a construct closely linked to Neuroticism) is the key feature of BPD. This hypothesis was revised to include traits of impulsivity as an additional risk factor (Crowell et al., 2010). It is the combination of dysregulated emotion and impulsive actions, with effects in turn on interpersonal relationships, that defines this disorder.

Thus, Linehan argued for a gene–environment "biosocial" model of BPD, suggesting that the environmental component in BPD consists largely of a failure by significant others to validate and contain intense emotions. She also hypothesized that problems with emotion regulation, affecting both its intensity and duration, are rooted in heritable traits—a view that has gained considerable empirical support (Knopik et al., 2017; Livesley et al., 1998). A failure to validate emotions can be considered a form of emotional neglect. A good body of research supports the conclusion that emotional invalidation plays a key role in BPD patients (Paris, 2020a).

Another, and rather popular, view of BPD sees its causes as deriving primarily from the long-term impact of childhood trauma. There is indeed a high frequency of histories of childhood trauma in these patients (Zanarini, 2000, 2005). There is also a high rate of PTSD (but still a minority) among BPD patients (Gunderson & Sabo, 1993). Those favoring a posttraumatic model of the disorder have been particularly impressed by the potential impact of childhood sexual abuse (CSA). Our own research team studied both females and males with BPD (Paris et al., 1994a, 1994b) and found that about a third of them had a history of CSA that went beyond a single incident. However, that leaves a majority without such a history.

It is quite another matter to propose that BPD is a form of PTSD. This attempt at reducing a complex disorder to a single cause does not concur with the evidence of research, and it fails to take personality into account. Once again, keep in mind that personality traits mediate and process the impact of environmental events. Moreover, it is a stretch to attribute all the features of a disorder, including emotion dysregulation and impulsivity, to adversities during childhood. In fact, the relationship between child abuse and BPD is not very consistent. In our research (Paris et al., 1994a, 1994b) and in work carried out by other investigators (Zanarini, 2000), while a significant minority had a history of CSA, the majority of those with the diagnosis did not report CSA. Studies that have reported a much higher rate have generally considered CSA as a single variable without considering its parameters. The result was an overestimation of frequency due to failing to exclude life events that did not involve physical contact, or events occurring during adolescence that involved peers (which do not carry the same implications or consequences as abuse by caretakers or family members).

This conclusion has been supported by meta-analyses. Fossati et al. (1999) found the effect size of CSA in relation to BPD to be .28. A more recent meta-analysis examining 97 clinical and community studies (Porter et al., 2020) found that 32% of BPD patients have a history of CSA, very similar to our own findings and those of other investigators who examined the parameters of abuse in detail.

If one compares patients with BPD to those with other mental disorders, then CSA is certainly more frequent. However, these are mean differences driven by a subgroup of BPD patients exposed to higher levels of adversity. But while patients with BPD do not always have a history of CSA, those who do tend to have both a severe and chronic course of BPD, as well as a higher frequency of suicide attempts (Soloff & Chiappetta, 2019). Thus, child abuse is an additional risk factor, but not the one or major cause of the disorder.

The childhood adversity that is most often reported in BPD patients is *emotional neglect*, which is described by the vast majority (Paris, 2020a). That is precisely what Linehan's theory would have predicted. Patients who have been abused will also have been neglected, in a clearly dysfunctional family environment and/or in one that fails to validate and understand the emotions of children. This helps explain why a multivariate analysis in a large community sample (Nash et al., 1993) found that family dysfunction accounted for most of the variance in psychopathology associated with CSA. This helps explain why emotional neglect is the most common factor promoting dysregulation. These kinds of environments are also the ones in which traumatic episodes are more likely to occur.

In summary, the attribution of causality to the relation between BPD and trauma, particularly CSA, is flawed and overly invested. What has been found can be summarized as follows:

1. A significant minority of BPD patients will have experienced CSA that involved physical contact.

2. CSA and other forms of childhood maltreatment (physical abuse, emotional abuse) make symptoms worse but do not predict BPD on their own.

3. Traumatic risk factors have a high co-occurrence with overall family dysfunction.

4. Children who experience CSA are also more likely to be emotionally neglected and invalidated.

5. CSA has a stronger effect on those who are temperamentally vulnerable.

These conclusions parallel a more general view that trauma does not consistently predict PTSD. Trauma also does not predict the development of a personality disorder.

Yet the drama of trauma tends to trump research evidence supporting a complex and multivariate pathway to mental disorders in general, and to PTSD in particular. However, those who support a trauma-focused model have found a way to redefine the problem by creating new categories that fail to recognize the power of personality traits and disorders.

THE DIAGNOSIS OF COMPLEX PTSD

Herman (1992) was the first to propose the diagnostic construct of complex posttraumatic stress disorder (CPTSD). The word "complex" is a little tricky. The theory is that repeated and multiple traumas, particularly in childhood, lead to outcomes that go beyond those of single traumas. Up to a point, that idea is consistent with the literature of the cumulative effects of adversities (Rutter et al., 2012).

Herman went on to argue that CSA, as well as multiple sexual assaults later in development, can lead to widespread personality problems including mood instability, somatization, dissociation, substance abuse, identity diffusion, self-harm, suicidality, and conflictual relationships. Thus, CPTSD is separated from ordinary PTSD on the grounds that the outcomes are more relational than symptomatic, more related to unstable mood and impulsivity than to the anxiety-driven picture of the classical disorder.

In DSM-5, no distinction is made between classical and complex PTSD. But in ICD-11, it is now listed as an official diagnosis (World Health Organization [WHO], 2019). Here is the ICD-11 definition of the disorder as described on the WHO website:

Complex post-traumatic stress disorder (complex PTSD) is a disorder that may develop following exposure to an event or series of events of an extremely threatening or horrific nature, most commonly prolonged or repetitive events from which escape is difficult or impossible (e.g., torture, slavery, genocide campaigns, prolonged domestic violence, repeated childhood sexual or physical abuse). All diagnostic requirements for PTSD are met. In addition, Complex PTSD is characterized by severe and persistent 1) problems in affect regulation; 2) beliefs about oneself as diminished, defeated or worthless, accompanied by feelings of shame, guilt or failure related to the traumatic event; and 3) difficulties in sustaining relationships and in feeling close to others. These symptoms cause significant impairment in personal, family, social, educational, occupational or other important areas of functioning.

This definition seems to offer a relabeling of BPD as CPTSD. It is a dangerously simple idea that tempts clinicians to search actively for episodes that are traumatic in the life histories of patients. That is to say, this search will be affected by a *confirmation bias*: If you are looking for trauma, you will be more likely to find it.

Some of the research supporting the CPTSD concept has been led by the University of London psychologist Chris Brewin. Over several decades, Brewin has been an opponent of the skeptics of recovered memory, and he has challenged the work of Elizabeth Loftus on this issue (Read & Lindsay, 1997). Brewin believes that memories can have a *dual representation* in the mind, and that one of these pathways is consistent with a mechanism of repression (Brewin & Andrews, 1998, 2017). Thus, the concept of CPTSD may make one sympathetic to ideas about repressed and recovered memories.

In a review paper produced by an ICD-11 committee that studied the evidence for this new diagnosis, Brewin et al. (2017) argued that CPTSD needs to be separated from PTSD, mainly because it describes mechanisms particular to repeated childhood trauma. The committee also developed a questionnaire to diagnose CPTSD (Karatzias et al., 2017) and used statistical methods (latent class analysis) to show that it is different from classical PTSD (Cloitre et al., 2014). Another latent class analysis (Frost et al., 2018) distinguished CPTSD from BPD due to a stronger relationship with a traumatic history. However, this is a rather circular argument: CPTSD is defined as based in trauma, while BPD is not.

In a review of this controversy, Ford and Courtois (2014) argued that while CPTSD overlaps with BPD, it does not do so often enough to justify considering it as a subtype of the personality disorder. Moreover, it is not at all clear, given the definition of CPTSD, what a case that met these criteria would look like without also meeting criteria for a personality disorder. BPD is a broader (albeit more heterogeneous) construct, and most people with BPD do not have PTSD.

Another problem is that research into differences between CPTSD and BPD has been conducted in populations exposed to trauma. But if trauma is not the primary cause of BPD, one will not find most affected patients in these populations. Moreover, symptoms and early life histories are insufficient to determine the validity of the disorder (Ford, 2020). Finally, as pointed out by Lehrner and Yehuda (2020), clinicians may come to believe that CPTSD responds to the same treatment methods as PTSD, a conclusion not justified by current research.

In spite of these problems, CPTSD is well on the way to becoming a popular diagnosis, even in North America, where few clinicians make regular use of the ICD-11 system. CPTSD has been promoted by academicians who specialize in PTSD, and this commitment can lead to what has been called "concept creep," the tendency to expand the definition of a construct. Finally, CPTSD may be favored by clinicians attracted by the greater simplicity of attribution of symptoms to trauma, but with a label that allows for discrepancies between exposure and outcome by describing clinical features as "complex." Some patients have become attached to this label, possibly because it puts the blame on other people for their problems.

Since the definition of CPTSD in ICD-11 describes problems in emotion regulation as well as difficulties in sustaining relationships or in feeling close to others, these criteria might be applied to a subgroup of BPD patients with prominent histories of severe childhood trauma. Yet patients can develop BPD without trauma, in spite of having almost identical symptoms to those who have been exposed to it. (This is the danger of seeing symptoms as having etiological meaning, as opposed to the effects of many different pathways to psychopathology.) Even among those BPD patients who are comorbid for PTSD, trauma is unlikely to explain the wide range of their problems with emotion regulation, impulsivity, and interpersonal relationships.

In an attempt to simplify a complex set of etiological pathways, the CPTSD construct removes the role of personality in personality disorder. Without an acknowledgment of interactions between heritable traits and a broader range of life experiences, making this diagnosis is misleading and can lead to approaches to psychotherapy that are less than ideal.

I would ask: If we already have a name for the clinical picture of BPD (described in thousands of research papers), and if research on BPD has demonstrated a large heritable component as well as defined environmental factors in its etiology, what is the point or renaming and reformulating the disorder? One reason may be that BPD seems to carry a stigma while CPTSD might not. BPD has long had a stigma (Aviram et al., 2006). Yet calling these problems by another name will not take them away. Whatever the cause of their disorder, BPD patients are stigmatized due to their chronic suicidality and out-of-control emotions. When you change the name of a disorder, you don't do much to remove stigma. Patients are no better understood or accepted in today's society when the names of their conditions have been changed. If we were to replace "BPD" with "CPTSD," we would leave the majority of these patients as orphans of the diagnostic system and compromise access to the evidence-based treatments that can reverse most of the effects of this personality disorder (Paris, 2020a).

It is understandable that clinicians want to avoid "blaming the victim," but CPTSD is a diagnosis that blames other people. That is the same bias discussed throughout this book, one that favors a focus on the nature of traumatic events and not on the people who experience them. At best, CTPSD defines a subgroup of BPD patients with a comorbidity that leads to a more severe course of illness.

Let's consider research evidence on patients who have both disorders. A community study (Zlotnick et al., 2006) compared patients with various personality disorders who either had or did not have PTSD. The findings were that the presence or absence of comorbid PTSD had no effect on the core construct of BPD in terms of its effects on emotions, impulsivity, and relationships.

Another community study, by Scheiderer et al. (2015), found that while about half of patients with BPD can be diagnosed with comorbid PTSD, only half of these cases derived from CSA, with the other half reflecting the effects of later traumatic events of various kinds (such as accidents, war, or violent confrontations). The most consistent histories in this population are of milder, less pathogenic experiences that cannot readily be classified as traumatic but are clearly neglectful (Zanarini et al., 2017).

Decades ago, Yehuda (1999, p. xiii) summed up the literature on personality and PTSD by noting that invoking trauma exposure as the primary etiological factor in PTSD may "spare victims the indignity of being misunderstood as 'neurotic' or constitutionally weak for succumbing to the effects of traumatic event." However, as noted by Miller et al. (2006, p. 374), "despite the clinical appeal of this position, the assumption that exposure to trauma is the primary etiological factor in PTSD has been contradicted by accumulating empirical evidence." Little has changed in the years since these papers were published.

Two decades ago, I reviewed research on PTSD and personality (Paris, 2000a) and came to the same conclusion. Thus, personality shapes response to the environment and is the main source of variability in responses to trauma. Most of the research concerns Neuroticism, which has also been called "negative emotionality" (Miller, 2003). The trait that governs a tendency to experience anxiety and depression is also one of the strongest predictors of PTSD. Patients with high Neuroticism trait respond more strongly to stress and also take longer to come back to baseline.

The emotional dysregulation that characterizes patients with BPD is also similar to Neuroticism, and this helps explain why these patients respond the way they do to traumatic events. It also helps explain why emotional neglect can be experienced as profoundly toxic and disruptive, sometimes leading to feelings of self-hatred.

The symptoms associated with a PTSD diagnosis are not specific to their triggers. They reflect a level of emotional vulnerability that leads people to develop a strong reaction to adversity. We can gain greater understanding of these pathways by framing them within personality trait profiles.

In BPD, the theory that emotion dysregulation is the key to understanding the disorder has now gained wide empirical support. (Paris, 2020a). Personality disorders arise from gene–environment interactions between heritable traits and environmental risks. Moreover, Linehan's (1993) focus on decreasing emotion dysregulation is often the main focus of therapy in BPD patients and has the most research support of any therapy for the disorder.

I am left with concern as to whether many BPD patients will be referred for therapies designed for classical PTSD and not for problematic personality traits. By focusing too much on trauma, CPTSD interferes with a broader understanding of the biopsychosocial roots of BPD, as well as with access to treatments that better reflect the current state of scientific knowledge.

Chapter 8

Treatment for Posttraumatic Stress Disorder

DOES POSTTRAUMATIC STRESS DISORDER REQUIRE TRAUMA-SPECIFIC PSYCHOTHERAPY?

We know from a vast research literature that psychotherapies are efficacious for a wide variety of psychological problems in a broad range of patients (Markham et al., 2021). Yet by and large, psychological interventions mainly help patients not due to specific interventions but rather to nonspecific *common factors*—that is, ingredients that can be found in all effective forms of treatment. That is why head-to-head comparisons of different evidence-based methods of therapy almost always find no difference in outcome (Wampold, 2001). This lack of difference has been called the "dodo bird verdict," after a scene in the book *Alice's Adventures in Wonderland* where the bird announces that all have won a race and that all shall have prizes. The most important common factors in therapy consist of the quality of the relationship, the therapeutic alliance, a high level of empathy, congruence with the patient's worldview, and the skill of the therapist in providing care. Decades ago, Frank and Frank (1991) argued that the most common element in effective treatment consists of providing hope and combating hopelessness.

Clinicians who do not know this literature may be prone to be impressed by claims to uniqueness from the hundreds of brand-name therapies on the market. This resembles the situation when pharmaceutical companies focus marketing on dissatisfied physicians by putting out a "me-too" drug that does not differ from those that are already available. Practitioners may want to try "the latest thing" in the hope that what is newest will be more effective. And as in the case of pharmaceuticals, there is money to be made from promoting psychotherapies, by attracting people to conferences and selling books. Many current therapies have easy-to-remember three- or four-letter acronyms; at times, it seems that evidence-based practice is trumped by acronym-based treatment.

Posttraumatic stress disorder (PTSD), with prominent symptoms related to traumatic experiences, has been a particular magnet for therapies that claim specificity. These methods aim to help patients process traumatic memories, overcome problematic thoughts and behaviors, and develop effective coping and interpersonal skills. Most of these treatments are either part of a package of cognitive-behavioral therapy (CBT) or derived from CBT.

The principle behind some of the best-studied interventions for PTSD is that by avoiding triggers, patients fail to extinguish conditioned responses to fear (Foa & Kozak, 1986). In this view, patients require reexposure to a traumatic memory in order to process it. That could be accomplished by reliving the experience in one's imagination under the supervision of a therapist who teaches the patient how to reduce the toxicity of these memories.

These concepts are the basis of *exposure therapy* (Rauch et al., 2012) or a variant called *prolonged exposure* (Rauch & Foa, 2006). ET was the first method of treatment for PTSD to gain support from clinical trials and still has the strongest evidence base. Its procedure involves retelling the traumatic event, followed by in vivo exposure to triggers, and then unpairing the memory from states of anxiety. Frueh et al. (2018, p. 178) summarized this literature: "At this point, variations on exposure therapy and cognitive therapy appear to be the primary efficacious psychotherapies for treating PTSD."

However, as pointed out by McNally (2007), a significant minority of patients do not benefit from exposure therapy. While proponents (e.g., Rauch et al., 2012), have dubbed exposure therapy a "gold standard," it does not necessarily yield better results than older methods.

It may be that efficacy depends largely on processing and contextualizing a trauma in one's mind, so that processing an experience need not require reexposure alone. In this view, efficacious methods focus less on reexperiencing the trauma than on reframing it, as in standard CBT. Some specialized methods such as *cognitive processing therapy* developed for rape victims (Resick & Schnicke, 1993) apply this model. In this way, therapy can target Neuroticism, and not just memories.

Let us now consider a currently popular method based on the recall and reprocessing of traumatic experiences: *eye movement desensitization and reprocessing* (EMDR; Shapiro, 1989). EMDR is widely used, has gained support from clinical trials, and has been recommended by National Institute for Clinical Excellence (2018) guidelines, as well as by a Cochrane report (Bisson et al., 2013). This form of treatment for PTSD has also gained substantial publicity. But like most therapies, while EMDR is superior to placebo or waiting list comparisons, it does not yield better results than other well-structured treatments (Chen et al., 2015). When comparative trials are carried out for psychotherapies of all kinds for mental disorders, that is the most common verdict (Wampold et al., 2010).

EMDR differs from exposure therapy primarily by its use of eye movements to guide patients in reexperiencing the traumatic event, again with the goal of taking the sting out of these memories. But while reprocessing memories is an element in most therapies for PTSD, there is no evidence that the use of a wand by a therapist to guide eye movements is necessary. This procedure could probably be called a gimmick. For that reason, EMDR may be no more specific to trauma than similar methods used by Franz Mesmer in the 18th century to guide people to undergo hypnosis (McNally, 1999).

In summary, systematic reviews and meta-analyses support the conclusion that EMDR is efficacious for PTSD but do not support the view that it has more specific and more powerful effects than other trauma-focused methods (Bisson et al., 2013; Chen et al., 2015; Seidler & Wagner, 2013). Enthusiasm for a specific method can shape research results, particularly when it is new, but effects may decline with time (Kagan, 1994, 1998). A well-known Dutch psychotherapy group (Cuijpers et al., 2020) reviewed 27 studies of EMDR and concluded that most suffered from publication bias. As summarized by Lohr et al. (2014, p. 292):

The scientific literature on EMDR supports several conclusions: (1) EMDR is an efficacious treatment for PTSD, (2) the efficacy of EMDR is comparable with that of trauma-focused CBT approaches such as [prolonged exposure], and (3) eye movements and other bilateral stimulation techniques appear to be unnecessary and do not uniquely contribute to clinical outcomes . . . EMDR offers few, if any, demonstrable advantages over competing evidence-based psychological treatments. Moreover, its theoretical model and purported primary active therapeutic ingredient are not scientifically supported.

Another problem with the "trauma-focused" therapies is the accuracy of memories of trauma. Engelhard et al. (2019) views the instability of accurate recall to be a limitation of all these methods. Traumatic memories, like other kinds of memories, tend to change each time they are recalled (McNally, 2012).

Trauma-focused cognitive-behavioral therapy (TF-CBT; Deblinger et al., 2006) also has evidential support from research. TF-CBT was originally designed for PTSD in maltreated children and adolescents and involved parents in family therapy. Its evidence base in clinical trials on this population is good, and it has been recommended both by the National Institute of Clinical Excellence (2018) and, with some reservations, by a Cochrane report (Bisson et al., 2013). But again, it has not been shown that TF-CBT is superior to standard treatments (Leenarts et al., 2013).

TF-CBT is now being used in adult populations, and it differs from standard CBT by adding a larger component of trauma processing. However, meta-analyses show either few differences (Ehlers et al., 2010) or no clinically significant differences (Wampold et al., 2010) from standard methods. In both National Institute of Clinical Excellence guidelines and the Cochrane report, while both TF-CBT and EMDR are considered efficacious, results were not strongly related to specific methods.

It is also worth keeping in mind that results depend on the comparison group. Much of the evidence for the specificity of trauma-focused therapies is based on comparisons between these methods and relatively weak forms of CBT, such as stress management. Almost any well-structured therapy tends to be better than "treatment as usual," which describes what goes on in clinics (but does not follow evidence-based protocols). Thus, there is insufficient evidence to conclude that either EMDR or TF-CBT is more efficacious than well-conducted standard CBT.

To conclude definitively that any of the more putatively specific interventions that therapists offer for patients with PTSD, such as exposure and processing of traumatic events, are specific, one would need to conduct a "dismantling study" in which specific elements are added or subtracted to determine what works and what does not. But dismantling is a lengthy and expensive procedure that is rarely carried out in psychotherapy research.

In summary, the empirical literature shows that PTSD responds to a variety of interventions and that common factors in treatment could account for most of the results. It remains to be determined whether a focus on remembering the details of a traumatic experience is crucial. Since standard CBT still has a large number of studies supporting its efficacy for PTSD (Kar, 2011), it might be considered a default option in practice. And over time, specific techniques developed as alternatives to common practices tend to be incorporated into more generic therapies. (This happened in my own field of personality disorders, where the emotion regulation strategies of dialectical behavior therapy [DBT] are now used by therapists of many persuasions.)

Keep in mind that posttraumatic symptoms are embedded in personality traits and interpersonal functioning. In this context, interpersonal therapy (IPT) takes a different approach from trauma-focused therapies or from standard CBT, emphasizing problems in current intimate relationships rather than in cognition and mental processing (Weissman et al., 2000). In one randomized clinical trial, PTSD patients were assigned to CBT or IPT and there was no difference in outcome (Markowitz et al., 2015). The authors of this study concluded that contrary to clinical opinion, exposure may not be a crucial element in the treatment of PTSD. While they did not compare IPT to trauma-focused therapies, one suspects that, once again, the "dodo bird verdict" might well have been triumphant.

Wampold (2019) has published an article called "A Smorgasbord of PTSD Treatments: What Does This Say About Integration?" His view is that the more treatment options are on the market, the more likely it is that they are doing the same thing. Moreover, even when methods claim uniqueness, they are probably integrative without quite acknowledging eclecticism. Wampold interprets the evidence as showing (p. 65) "that all treatments for PTSD are approximately equally effective and that the evidence for the mechanisms of change underlying the various treatments is weak."

Another topic that has attracted attention in the research literature, as well as among the general public, concerns the question as to whether early interventions can protect people against PTSD. Twenty years ago, there was a fad for "debriefing" sessions after traumatic exposure, and for a time, counselors would race to the scene soon after tragedies (such as terrorist attacks). However, research later showed that such interventions are not effective and may actually be counterproductive, by making people talk about events before they are ready to do so (Ehlers & Clark, 2003; McNally et al., 2003). Thus, while some have suggested that immediate interventions with a single session provided to people exposed to trauma may actually prevent the development of PTSD (Mitchell & Everly, 2000), the evidence does not support that conclusion. In fact, meta-analyses have shown that this method, called "critical incident stress debriefing," usually has little effect and may even make posttraumatic symptoms worse (van Emmerik et al., 2002). It seems likely that this type of intervention may have done a good deal of harm. Even so, one can read in the media about counselors being called to the scene of all kinds of traumatic events.

A related question is to what extent "triggers" related to traumatic memories need to be avoided to prevent PTSD symptoms from reappearing. But that may be still another myth we have to contend with. Jones et al. (2020), in a large sample of trauma survivors, found no such effect. This has not prevented the academic world from fearing reactions to purported triggering among their students. I have attended lectures at my own university in which, due to the raising of controversial issues, it was announced that counselors were available at the back of the hall if anyone in the audience was upset by the presentation. This scenario could be one of the worst outcomes of the culture of PTSD.

Finally, PTSD is not, like congestive heart failure, a distinct category of disease with distinct mechanisms. It is a syndrome that can vary from a relatively normal reaction to a stressful circumstance to a debilitating disorder. We should therefore not be surprised that there is no single or definitive treatment for this disorder. One can therefore envisage a stepped-care approach in which less extensive and less specific treatments are tried first, leaving the more complex interventions for a later step in those who do not benefit.

PHARMACOTHERAPY FOR PTSD

Not everyone with PTSD benefits from psychotherapy. For this reason, Bisson et al. (2020) recommended that pharmacotherapy be kept in reserve as a second-line treatment. A Cochrane report (Stein et al., 2000) found value for the use of specific serotonin uptake inhibitors in this patient population, and two agents in this class (sertraline and paroxetine) have been approved by the U.S. Food and Drug Administration. However, while this level of evidence is sufficient for U.S. government approval, it is not known whether patients need to stay on these agents for long periods, or whether positive findings derive from the nonspecific effects of antidepressants on anxiety (Alexander, 2012). As in the psychotherapy literature, lack of specificity tends to be more the exception than the rule.

Another source of nonspecificity derives from diagnosis. Clinicians have been using DSMs for so long that they mistakenly assume that psychiatric diagnoses are scientifically valid categories. That is far from being the case (Paris, 2020d). The manuals we use describe syndromes, not diseases, which overlap so much that some have suggested replacing all categories of mental disorder with dimensional scores (Kotov et al., 2017).

PTSD is no exception. It is a variant of a group of internalizing disorders characterized by high Neuroticism, and it has a very high comorbidity (50%) with major depression and anxiety disorders (Flory & Yehuda, 2015). Thus, antidepressants may target "comorbid" mood symptoms and/or have a nonspecific effect in reducing anxiety without removing core posttraumatic symptoms. It is possible that psychotherapy has more lasting effects (Lancaster et al., 2016). What is missing from the literature, however, are follow-up studies to determine whether improvement with either method of treatment remains stable after treatment ends (Bradley et al., 2005). That is a general problem with treatment research. And it is particularly important in PTSD, since more severe cases can go on to chronicity.

Finally, a Cochrane review (Hetrick et al., 2010) found no evidence for the efficacy of combined psychotherapy and antidepressant treatment. This conclusion has evidently not been taken into account in practice, given that this combination is what most PTSD patients currently receive.

HOW THERAPY HELPS—AND WHY IT DOESN'T ALWAYS HELP

I have expressed doubt about the need for a routine prescription of specialized therapies for PTSD. A number of features of standard CBT account for its effectiveness in this population. As summarized by Kar (2011, p. 177):

> Various cognitive distortions are seen in PTSD, depending on the traumatic experience and the nature of the psychological state of the person. Common cognitive distortions include perceiving the world as dangerous, seeing oneself as powerless or inadequate, or feeling guilty about outcomes that could not have been prevented . . . PTSD is associated with negative beliefs about self that may influence self-esteem and interpersonal relationships. PTSD often co-occurs with depression, and they may share common risk factors. One possible common cognitive risk factor is hopelessness.

These comments focus on the basic elements of any CBT intervention and echo the literature on the role of common factors in therapy. Given the vast literature supporting the efficacy of CBT for a wide range of diagnoses, it should not be surprising that it also works for PTSD. Yet, as Kar (2011) acknowledges, about half of PTSD patients fail to respond to psychotherapy. He views this problem as most likely due to *comorbidities*. But these additional diagnoses need not be thought of as separate from PTSD, but rather as part of a larger pattern of vulnerability to distress that increases severity.

It is not surprising that the most common comorbidities of PTSD are mood and anxiety disorders (Knowles et al., 2019), given the symptomatic overlap between all these diagnoses. Perhaps the most problematic clinical issue is comorbidity with substance use disorders. Patients with PTSD have been shown to be up to 14 times more likely than patients without PTSD to have a substance use disorder (McCauley et al., 2012). This relationship could be due to self-medication of PTSD symptoms, but it is also possible that substance use disorder precedes the onset of PTSD, and it may also be associated with a tendency to engage in high-risk behaviors.

As discussed in Chapter 7, another significant comorbidity, and one that is often ignored, is personality disorder. For example, there is strong evidence for a relationship between PTSD and border-line personality disorder (BPD). Even if such cases are in the minority, they are common, both in clinical samples (Gunderson & Sabo, 1993) and in community populations (Pagura et al., 2010). Thus, individuals with comorbid PTSD and BPD were also much more likely than individuals with BPD alone and individuals with PTSD alone to have mood, anxiety, and substance use disorders. Personality disorders other than BPD are even more common. In a population of combat veterans (Bollinger et al., 2000), the most frequent personality disorder diagnoses were avoidant (47.2%), paranoid (46.2%), obsessive-compulsive (28.3%), and antisocial (15.1%).

An additional diagnosis of personality disorder in patients with PTSD has clinical implications. It usually means that in addition to posttraumatic symptoms, a patient has problems with mood regulation, impulse control, identity, a sense of self, and close relationships. These problems may also respond to treatment originally designed for PTSD.

TREATING PTSD IN THE CONTEXT OF PERSONALITY DISORDER

In the history of psychotherapy, treatments, ranging from psychoanalysis to the latest acronym-based therapy, have often claimed to be either definitive in their effects or specific to particular symptoms. But research shows that effective therapy can be based on many different theories and practices. Most people get better if they feel understood and receive useful feedback.

I have no problem accepting that trauma-focused therapies work, but we cannot say for sure that an emphasis on emotional processing of memories is a necessary ingredient. The risk may be less in time-limited therapy; therapists usually treat patients briefly for a few months, avoiding the dangers of regression in open-ended treatment and maximizing a focus on autonomy, confidence, and hopefulness.

My concern relates more to more severe cases, in which extended courses of therapy may be offered to patients with both PTSD and BPD. Since BPD is my subspecialty, many of the patients I see do have significant histories of trauma. Yet something less than half of BPD patients report childhood sexual abuse, while the vast majority describe a narrative of emotional neglect (Paris, 2020a). Moreover, many of the traumas they do report occur in adolescence, a stage at which BPD can already be recognized. Thus, adversities that are consequences of BPD can be counted as potential causes.

Although the criteria required for a diagnosis of BPD are now better known, clinicians tend to be impressed by traumatic histories. The result is that many of these patients will receive a PTSD (or complex PTSD) diagnosis. In that case, they may receive therapy that focuses on the past and not on the present. But these patients have serious problems in their current life related to emotion dysregulation and impulsivity (suicide attempts, self-harm, and substance use) as well as highly problematic intimate relationships.

Another wrinkle in this story is that BPD patients have an unusual number of traumatic experiences as *adults*. Specifically, they often tend to become victims of interpersonal violence (Zanarini et al., 1999). This is partly due to their tendency to choose problematic partners, partly due to their impulsivity, and partly due to a strong need to be another person as a way of regulating emotions. For example, BPD patients are at risk for being raped, and at least some of these incidents are related to substance abuse. It is not so much, as some have claimed, a matter of repeating trauma but rather of getting into dangerous situations and not having the skills to cope with danger. Finally, since patients with BPD score high on Neuroticism (Samuel & Widiger, 2008), they have less ability to be resilient after trauma.

In the Canadian province where I work, we have universal health insurance for care by physicians, but psychologists are poorly covered (if at all). But the government has created a program to provide insurance for victims of violence, called *Indemnisation des Victimes d'Actes Criminels* (IVAC). The result is that if you were beaten up by your boyfriend and if the police were called and charges were laid, you will be eligible for free weekly therapy lasting about 1 to 2 years. I have no data on the results of this well-intentioned program, but I have the impression from some patients who have been in it that the focus is almost entirely on the processing of traumatic memories, especially from childhood. Moreover, this approach is being used in patients who are highly dysfunctional and who have no lack of current problems.

Trauma-focused treatment contrasts with my clinic's short-term BPD program, which I have described in a previous book (Paris, 2017) and which has been supported by effectiveness data (Laporte et al., 2018). Most of our treatments are brief (3 months) and oriented to current functioning, not to the past. We do listen to trauma histories, but we put more emphasis on regulating emotion, controlling impulsivity, improving relationships, and getting back to work or school. This approach is also consistent with an understanding that trauma is not the only cause of PTSD, and that both PTSD and personality disorders require a biopsychosocial treatment model.

PSYCHOTHERAPY, PTSD, AND PHILOSOPHY

The most effective treatments for PTSD are almost all, in one way or the other, derived from the principles of CBT. In its present form, cognitive therapy is a relatively recent development that first appeared about 60 years ago. Yet its roots go back 2,000 years, to Stoic philosophy (Robertson & Codd, 2019). Both Albert Ellis and Aaron Beck acknowledged their debt to these ancient thinkers. CBT, especially in its "third wave" (Hayes & Hoffman, 2017), as in Acceptance and Commitment Therapy (ACT; Hayes, 2012), is consistent with Stoicism. This also applies to DBT, which makes use of some principles of classical Buddhism. This is most apparent in the concept of mindfulness (training one's attention to remain in the present moment; Segal et al., 2013) and in concepts such as "radical acceptance" (Linehan, 1993; moving from an orientation to the past to one that focuses on the future).

Stoicism emerged in the third century BCE, and these ideas are associated with Greek and Roman philosophers such as Zeno,

Epictetus, Seneca, and Marcus Aurelius. One of its central principles was used by Shakespeare when Hamlet remarks, "There is nothing either good or bad but thinking makes it so." That sounds quite a bit like CBT.

What are the key elements of Stoic philosophy? Many of them concern how people deal with adversity in life. A Stoic is advised to cultivate four cardinal virtues: wisdom, morality, courage, and moderation. The philosophy does not correspond to the way the term is used today, describing a suppression of emotion. Rather, it more like CBT or the famous Serenity Prayer by Reinhold Niebuhr: "God, grant me the serenity to accept the things I cannot change, the courage to change the things I can, and the wisdom to know the difference." Thus, Stoicism advises us to accept what we cannot change (e.g., death or loss) and to focus our energies on what we can change (e.g., feelings of unbearable grief and hopelessness).

With these principles in mind, I worry that trauma-focused therapies may focus on the wrong issues. What I am concerned about is the potential for missing the broader context of PTSD. But in view of the central role of common factors, most therapies help patients even when their theoretical basis is problematic.

Another philosophical issue that needs to be considered in relation to therapies for trauma is the debate between free will and determinism. In working as a psychotherapist, almost everything I do with patients assumes the reality of free will. If I thought that they had no choice but to suffer, there would no point in working with them.

No matter how badly traumatized people are, they can choose agency over victimhood. This is the lesson I draw from research on resilience. There are limits to this freedom—some of the most badly traumatized Romanian orphans will never be able to have fully normal lives. But for most circumstances in life, freedom to choose is a function of the complex evolution of the brain and mind. Determinism may be a correct view for nonliving things, or for the behavior of microorganisms, but is not a good model for human beings. As the American philosopher Daniel Dennett (2003) nicely put it, free will exists and freedom evolves. This is why psychotherapy for people with PTSD should not be trauma-focused but should focus on the person who experiences distress.

IMPLICATIONS FOR CLINICAL PRACTICE

One of the recurring themes of PTSD research has been the contrast between two perspectives (Grob & Horwitz, 2010). In the first, the focus is on the characteristics of the trauma itself, which is assumed to be capable of producing symptoms in almost any person. In the second, the focus is on individual differences in vulnerability to trauma.

This book has underlined the second perspective. The idea that mental health depends not on what we experience, but rather on how we process and understand our lives, has a long history. It can be traced back to philosophies such as Buddhism and Stoicism. This is the same idea that underlies CBT, which teaches people how to manage emotions associated with adverse life events. In other words, clinicians need not see adversities as unbuffered but should rather assume that a psychological immune system can be strengthened by interventions. People who develop PTSD can be taught to be more resilient.

The wide influence of the PTSD construct threatens to make victimhood into an ideology and a cultural icon. This trend is particularly apparent in attitudes that have been common in the "recovery movement" (Kaminer, 1992). But clinicians who follow that script run the danger of reinforcing a process in which victimhood becomes a central part of one's identity. The problem is that seeing oneself as a victim tends to support chronicity. Maintaining a focus on trauma rather than functioning can reinforce this self-image. This may be particularly important in PTSD, since narratives of victimization can sometimes dominate the discourse of psychotherapy. Instead, treatment can aim to restore a sense of *agency* (Knox, 2011).

I am in no way suggesting that clinicians should fail to acknowledge and explore histories of trauma. Patients need to tell their stories and have them validated. But they need not be viewed as victims of circumstance. A better way to look at them is as survivors, who, in spite of a traumatic past, are capable of resilience—moving on and getting a life.

Chapter 9

Summary and Conclusions

A BIOPSYCHOSOCIAL MODEL OF POSTTRAUMATIC STRESS DISORDER

Posttraumatic stress disorder (PTSD) is a complex syndrome with many causes and is not accounted for by trauma alone. Like other mental disorders, its etiology is biopsychosocial, requiring an interactive and complex model. This helps explain why most people exposed to traumatic events do not develop PTSD. Innate vulnerability factors linked to personality trait profiles modulate exposure and sensitivity to trauma. Those with high levels of Neuroticism, driven in part by genetic factors and in part by exposure to previous adversities, are most likely to develop symptoms. The extent to which predispositions are activated depends on stressful events— not on single stressors, but on the cumulative effects of multiple adverse events. This mechanism is a kind of kindling effect similar to that seen in recurrent depression (Monroe & Harkness, 2005). Finally, social factors can either be protective or increase the risk of sequelae.

All these factors play a role in the etiology of PTSD, varying from individual to individual in their strength. However, even when all risks are combined, they still fail to explain most of the outcome variance. As research progresses, we may well discover other risk and protective factors influencing the likelihood of developing PTSD after exposure to trauma. But while models similar to the one presented here have been suggested by others (McNally, 2012), additional work is needed to support their validity.

The problem for researchers is that since patients in clinical samples were already vulnerable to PTSD, biological predispositions can be ignored while correlations with psychosocial factors tend to be exaggerated. One way to get around this difficulty would be to conduct prospective community studies, ideally in twin samples to control for genetic effects. Large-scale community samples would also allow for conducting multivariate analyses of risk and protective factors, an approach consistent with the multidimensional nature of PTSD.

Yet since this would be a very expensive way of studying PTSD, very few studies of this kind have ever been launched or published. Even in the large-scale E-Risk study that prospectively followed up twins, while some form of trauma during development was ubiquitous (Fisher et al., 2015), data on PTSD as an outcome have not yet been published, possibly due to a low prevalence in nonclinical populations.

The greatest value of prospective longitudinal designs would be to measure interactions between predispositions present prior to traumatic exposure with stressful events. At the same time, one could determine how positive personality traits increase resilience to trauma. Moreover, prospective research would not depend on recall and could allow for more accurate measurements of trauma severity. A protocol for this kind of study, using a biopsychosocial model to predict PTSD, has been published (Wafa et al., 2019), and we can await its findings.

To shed light on social risk factors, more cross-cultural studies of PTSD are needed to determine how this disorder is related to traditional and modern societies. Research is also needed to determine whether variations in prevalence occur among subcultures within our own society.

CLINICAL IMPLICATIONS OF A BIOPSYCHOSOCIAL MODEL

Applying a biopsychosocial model to the understanding of PTSD has many useful clinical implications. PTSD is not a discrete category of illness, and it is not caused by trauma alone. Patients with this diagnosis do not necessarily need to be treated by trauma-focused interventions. Successful cognitive processing of a stressful experience may be sufficient for recovery from acute symptoms. The treatment of PTSD could be modified to focus more on thinking patterns rooted in personality traits. That approach has long been a basis for cognitive therapy. However, whether a more generic approach can yield the same success in patients with chronic PTSD symptoms associated with comorbid conditions such as substance use and personality disorder is more doubtful.

Another clinical implication of a broader model is that disorders with a complex etiology require complex and multimodal treatment. That almost involves psychotherapy, which has the strongest evidence base as a treatment for PTSD. Another advantage of psychotherapy is that it can modify Neuroticism without the risks of long-term pharmacological treatment. Yet while pharmacotherapy retains a role as an adjunct to psychotherapy, treating patients with drugs alone is less likely to be successful. Unfortunately, psychotherapy for any mental disorder is much more difficult to access than pharmacotherapy. Talking therapy is resource-intensive, even in government-funded systems like the Veterans Administration in the United States or the National Health Service in the United Kingdom. For this reason, it may not always be available. The result is that many patients with PTSD are left only with access to checkups and prescriptions.

Finally, treatment based on a biopsychosocial model can be more forward-looking, as opposed to models that focus on the past. Patients would be encouraged to accept that the past cannot be changed, but that they can change their current life with an eye on the future.

MYTHS VERSUS EVIDENCE ABOUT TRAUMA

In the Introduction to this book, I listed 10 myths of trauma. I will now summarize my conclusions about them.

1. Trauma has become a catchword for many kinds of adverse experiences, yet this is a construct that needs to be more narrowly and precisely defined.
   Understanding PTSD requires a narrower definition of trauma. There is little doubt that rape and physical assault qualify as traumatic. However, some researchers and many clinicians have scored all kinds of adverse experience in life, from family breakdown to job loss, as qualifying as a traumatic stressor. This leads to overdiagnosis and to defining a clinical population that is too heterogeneous to be prescribed treatments that are specific for their problems.

2. Traumatic events have always been a part of human life, and most people are significantly resilient to adversity.

   The ubiquity of resilience is one of the most consistent findings in the trauma literature.

3. While trauma is necessary for PTSD, it is not sufficient. Exposure to trauma is only one cause of PTSD, and not necessarily the most important one. The disorder can only be understood in a biopsychosocial model, taking into account genetic vulnerability, personality trait profiles, previous adversities, and levels of social support.

   This book has reviewed a vast and complex literature showing that PTSD cannot be understood without considering interactions between multiple risk factors.

4. Trauma has often become a political issue that interferes with unbiased scientific study of its effects.

   Examples of the political nature of PTSD are far too many to list. Suffice it to say that anyone who challenges current diagnosis and practice in this population should be prepared for a hostile response.

5. The concept of repressed and recovered memories of traumatic events is scientifically invalid.

   This fad is fortunately less influential than it once was. The science is clear, and most knowledgeable therapists have never believed in it.

6. The wide comorbidity of PTSD, particularly when symptoms are chronic, means that it cannot be considered as a specific category with a specific treatment, and that treatment for patients should be broadly biopsychosocial.

   As I have documented, only a minority of PTSD patients have only one disorder. It does not make sense to focus on trauma when personality disorders and substance use disorder are also present.

7. Complex PTSD is a new diagnosis but is a problematic construct, given that most of its features can be better explained by personality disorders.

   The use of this new diagnosis offers an alternative for those who do not recognize the importance of personality, personality disorder, or the biological roots of response to life events. It is probably easier to focus on traumatic events than on current skills and functioning. However, diagnosing complex PTSD, and focusing almost entirely on trauma, may not be beneficial to patients.

8. Several evidence-based methods of treatment for PTSD have been developed, but their effectiveness is no greater than that of standard cognitive-behavioral therapy.

   You don't have to undertake advanced training to treat PTSD patients.

9. Understanding experiences of trauma has a place in the treatment of PTSD, but an excessive focus on memory processing can be a mistake.

   Spending precious time in therapy on the past may be done at the expense of problems in the present.

10. An excessive focus on trauma narratives can work against the interests of patients by encouraging victimhood instead of a sense of competence and agency.

    This is the dark side of well-intentioned psychotherapy. While patients may prefer to identify themselves as victims, doing so could encourage chronicity.

RECOMMENDATIONS

PTSD is a clinically important syndrome, but its scope has undergone concept creep, expanding well beyond what the evidence shows. The drama of traumatic events and the wish to focus on them in treatment have misled a generation of clinicians. If these theories were correct, one might expect to see a reduction of the prevalence of PTSD. Just the opposite has occurred, as PTSD has been used to describe a very wide variety of disorders in which trauma is only one of many risk factors.

These myths of trauma have not led to great benefit for patients. It is likely that relatively simple cases exist in which a single episode of trauma leads to psychopathology in those who are vulnerable. But the reification and expansion of PTSD have done a disservice to those who carry biological, psychological, and social factors and who suffer from a range of disorders, including depression, anxiety, substance use, and personality disorders.

Clinicians need to recognize the impact of trauma, but they also need to place it in a larger context. To accomplish this goal requires different ways of thinking that can navigate multivariate pathways and causal complexity.

REFERENCES

Afifi, T. O., Asmundson, G. J., Taylor, S., & Jang, K. L. (2010). The role of genes and environment on trauma exposure and posttraumatic stress disorder symptoms: A review of twin studies. *Clinical Psychology Review, 30*, 101–112.

Alexander, W. (2012). Pharmacotherapy for post-traumatic stress disorder in combat veterans. *Pharmacy and Therapeutics, 37*, 32–38.

Alford, C. F. (2016). *Trauma, culture, and PTSD*. Palgrave MacMillan.

Allen, M. T., Myers, C. E., Beck, K. D., Pang, K. C., & Servaituis, R. J. (2019). Inhibited personality temperaments translated through enhanced avoidance and associative learning increase vulnerability for PTSD. *Frontiers in Psychology, 10*, 496–501.

Amado, B. G., Fernandez, R. A., & Herraiz, A. (2015). Psychological injury in victims of child sexual abuse: A meta-analytic review. *Psychosocial Intervention, 24*, 49–62.

American Psychiatric Association. (1952). *Diagnostic and statistical manual of mental disorders* (1st ed.). American Psychiatric Publishing.

American Psychiatric Association. (1968). *Diagnostic and statistical manual of mental disorders* (2nd ed.). American Psychiatric Publishing.

American Psychiatric Association. (1980). *Diagnostic and statistical manual of mental disorders* (3rd ed.). American Psychiatric Publishing.

American Psychiatric Association. (1987). *Diagnostic and statistical manual of mental disorders* (3rd ed., revised). American Psychiatric Publishing.

American Psychiatric Association. (1994). *Diagnostic and statistical manual of mental disorders* (4th ed.). American Psychiatric Publishing.

American Psychiatric Association. (2013). *Diagnostic and statistical manual of mental disorders* (5th ed.). American Psychiatric Publishing.

Amstadter, A., Aggen, S., Knudsen, G., Reichborn-Kjennerud, T., & Kendler, K. (2012). A population-based study of familial and individual-specific environmental contributions to traumatic event exposure and posttraumatic stress disorder symptoms in a Norwegian twin sample. *Twin Research and Human Genetics, 15,* 656–662.

Andreasen, N. (1995). Posttraumatic stress disorder: Psychology, biology and the Manichaean warfare between false dichotomies. *American Journal of Psychiatry, 152,* 963–965.

Anokhin, A. P., Grant, J. D., Mulligan, R. C., & Heath, A. C. (2015). The genetics of impulsivity: Evidence for the heritability of delay discounting. *Biological Psychiatry, 77,* 887–894.

Armour, C., Fried, E. K., Deserno, M. K., Tsai, J., & Pietrzak, R. H. (2017). A network analysis of DSM-5 posttraumatic stress disorder symptoms and correlates in U.S. military veterans. *Journal of Anxiety Diseases, 45,* 4959.

Auxéméry, Y. (2012). Posttraumatic stress disorder (PTSD) as a consequence of the interaction between an individual genetic susceptibility, a traumatogenic event and a social context. *L'Encephale, 38,* 373–380.

Aviram, R. B., Brodsky, B. S., & Stanley, B. (2006). Borderline personality disorder, stigma, and treatment implications. *Harvard Review of Psychiatry, 14,* 249–256.

Baldwin, J. R., Arsenault, L., & Caspi, A. (2019). Adolescent victimization and self-injurious thoughts and behaviors: A genetically sensitive cohort study. *Journal of the American Academy of Child & Adolescent Psychiatry, 58,* 506–513.

Barel, E., Van IJzendoorn, M. H., Sagi-Schwartz, A., & Bakermans-Kranenburg, M. J. (2010). Surviving the Holocaust: A meta-analysis of the long-term sequelae of a genocide. *Psychological Bulletin, 136,* 677–698.

Bartlett, F. C. (1932). *Remembering: A study in experimental and social psychology.* Cambridge University Press.

Bass, E., & Davis, L. (1994). *The courage to heal: A guide for women survivors of child sexual abuse.* Harper and Row.

Beck, A. T., Davis, D., & Freeman, A. (2015). *Cognitive therapy of personality disorders* (3rd ed.). Guilford.

Bellet, B., Jones, P. J., & McNally, R. J. (2018). Trigger warning: Empirical evidence ahead. *Journal of Behavior Therapy & Experimental Psychiatry, 61,* 131–141.

Belsky, J., Caspi, A., Moffitt, T., & Poulton, R. (2020). *The origins of you: How childhood shapes later life.* Harvard University Press.

Belsky, J., & Pluess, M. (2009). The nature (and nurture?) of plasticity in early human development. *Perspectives in Psychological Science, 4,* 345–351.

Benjet, C., Bromet, E., Karam, E. G., Kessler, R. C., McLaughlin, K. A., Ruscio, A. M., Shahly, V., Stein, D. J., Petukhova, M., Hill, E., Alonso, J., Atwoli, L., Bunting, B., Bruffaerts, R., Caldas-de-Almeida, J. M., de Girolamo, G., Florescu, S., Gureje, O., Huang, Y., . . . Koenen, K. C. (2016). The epidemiology of traumatic event exposure worldwide: Results from the World Mental Health Survey Consortium. *Psychological Medicine, 46,* 327–343.

Bentall, R. (2003). *Madness explained: Psychosis and human nature.* Allen Lane.

Bernstein, E., & Putnam, F. (1986). Development, reliability, and validity of a dissociation scale. *Journal of Nervous and Mental Disease, 124,* 727–737.

Berntsen, D., & Rubin, D. C. (2007). When a trauma becomes a key to identity:
Enhanced integration of trauma memories predicts posttraumatic stress disorder symptoms. *Applied Cognitive Psychology, 21,* 417–431.

Bisson, J., Roberts, N. P., Andrew, M., Cooper, R., & Lewis, C. (2013). Psychological
therapies for chronic post-traumatic stress disorder (PTSD) in adults. *Cochrane
Database of Systematic Reviews, 12*(12), CD003388.

Bodkin, A., Pope, H. G., Delke, M. J., & Hudson, J. I. (2007). Is PTSD caused by
traumatic stress? *Journal of Anxiety Disorders, 21,* 176–182.

Bollinger, A. S., Riggs, D. S., Blake, D. D., & Ruzek, J. I. (2000). Prevalence of personality disorders among combat veterans with posttraumatic stress disorder.
Journal of Traumatic Stress, 13, 255–270.

Borsboom, D., & Cramer, A. O. J. (2013). Network analysis: An integrative approach
to the structure of psychopathology. *Annual Review of Clinical Psychology, 9,*
91–121.

Bowlby, J. (1969). *Attachment.* Hogarth.

Bowman, M., & Yehuda, R. (2004). Risk factors and the adversity-stress model. In
G. M. Rosen (Ed.), *Posttraumatic stress disorder: Issues and controversies* (pp. 39–
61). Wiley.

Boyce, C. A., & Maholmes, V. (2013). Attention to the neglected: Prospects for research on child neglect for the next decade. *Child Maltreatment, 18,* 65–68.

Bradley, R., Green, J., Dutra, L., & Westen, D. (2005). A multidimensional meta-
analysis of psychotherapy for PTSD. *American Journal of Psychiatry, 164,*
214–227.

Brady, K. T., Killeen, T. K., Brewerton, T., & Lucerini, S. (2000). Comorbidity of
psychiatric disorders and posttraumatic stress disorder. *Journal of Clinical
Psychiatry, 61*(Suppl. 7), 22–32.

Bremner, J. D., Randall, P., Scott, T. M., Bronen, R. A., Seibyl, J. P., Southwick, S.
M., Delaney, R. C., McCarthy, G., Charney, D. S., & Innis, R. B. (1995). MRI-
based measurement of hippocampal volume in patients with combat-related
posttraumatic stress disorder. *American Journal of Psychiatry, 152,* 973–981.

Breslau, N., Chilcoat, H. D., Kessler, R. C., & Davis, G. C. (1999). Previous exposure
to trauma and PTSD effects of subsequent trauma: Results from the Detroit
Area Survey of Trauma. *American Journal of Psychiatry, 156,* 902–907.

Breslau, N., Davis, G. C., Andreski, P., & Peterson, E. (1991). Traumatic events and
posttraumatic stress disorder in an urban population of young adults. *Archives of
General Psychiatry, 48,* 216–222.

Breslau, N., Kessler, R., Chilcoat, H. D., Schultz, L. R., Davis, G. C., & Andreski, P.
(1998). Trauma and posttraumatic stress disorder in the community: The 1996
Detroit area survey of trauma. *Archives of General Psychiatry, 55,* 626–632.

Breslau, N., & Schultz, L. (2013). Neuroticism and post-traumatic stress disorder: A prospective investigation. *Psychological Medicine, 43,* 1697–1702.

Breslau, N., Wilcox, H. C., Storr, C., Lucia, V. C., & Anthony, J. C. (2004). Trauma exposure and posttraumatic stress disorder: A study of youths in urban America. *Journal of Urban Health, 81,* 530–544.

Brewin, C. R., & Andrews, B. (1998). Recovered memories of trauma: Phenomenology and cognitive mechanisms. *Clinical Psychology Review, 18,* 949–970.

Brewin, C. R., & Andrews, B. (2017). False memories of childhood abuse. *Psychologist, 30,* 48–52.

Brewin, C. R., Cloitre, M., Hyland, P., Shevlin, M., Maercker, A., Bryant, R. A., Humayun, A., Jones, L. M., Kagee, A., Rousseau, C., Somasundaram, D., Suzuki, Y., Wessely, S., Ommeren, M., & Reed, G. M. (2017). A review of current evidence regarding the ICD-11 proposals for diagnosing PTSD and complex PTSD. *Clinical Psychology Review, 58,* 1–15.

Bromet, E., Karam, E., Koenen, K., Stein, D. (Eds.). (2018). *Trauma and posttraumatic stress disorder: Global perspectives from the WHO World Mental Health Surveys.* Cambridge University Press.

Browne, A., & Finkelhor, D. (1986). Impact of child sexual abuse: A review of the research. *Psychological Bulletin, 99,* 66–77.

Bryant, R. A. (2019). Post-traumatic stress disorder: A state-of-the-art review of evidence and challenges. *World Psychiatry, 18,* 259–269.

Bryant, R. A., & Harvey, A. G. (1998). Relationship between acute stress disorder and posttraumatic stress disorder following mild traumatic brain injury. *American Journal of Psychiatry, 155,* 625–629.

Burri, A., & Maercker, A. (2014). Differences in prevalence rates of PTSD in various European countries explained by war exposure, other trauma and cultural value orientation. *BMC Research Notes, 7,* 407.

Buss, D. (Ed.). (2005). *The handbook of evolutionary psychology.* Wiley.

Campbell, B., & Manning, J. (2018). *The rise of victimhood culture.* Palgrave MacMillan.

Caspi, A., McClay, J., Moffitt, T. E., Mill, J., Martin, J., Craig, I. W., Taylor, A., & Poulton, R. (2002). Role of genotype in the cycle of violence in maltreated children. *Science, 297,* 851–854.

Caspi, A., Moffitt, T. E., Newman, D. L., & Silva, P. A. (1996). Behavioral observations at age 3 years predict adult psychiatric disorders. *Archives of General Psychiatry, 53,* 1033–1039.

Caspi, A., Sugden, K., Moffitt, T. E., Taylor, A., Craig, I. W., Harrington, H., McClay, J., Mill, J., Martin, J., Braithwaite, A., & Poulton, R. (2003). Influence of life stress on depression: Moderation by a polymorphism in the 5-HTT gene. *Science, 301,* 386–389.

Cassidy, J., & Shaver, P. R. (Eds.). (2016). *Handbook of attachment: Theory, research and clinical aspects* (3rd ed.). Guilford.

Chen, G., Hu, M., & Liang, X. (2015). Eye movement desensitization and reprocessing versus cognitive-behavioral therapy for adult posttraumatic stress disorder: Systematic review and meta-analysis. *Journal of Nervous and Mental Disease, 203,* 443–451.

Chen, L. P., Murad, M. H., Paras, M. L., & Colbenson, K. M. (2010). Sexual abuse and lifetime diagnosis of psychiatric disorders: Systematic review and meta-analysis. *Mayo Clinic Procedings, 85,* 618–629.

Chiu, M., Amartey, A., Wang, X., Vigod, S., & Kurdyak, P. (2020). Trends in objectively measured and perceived mental health and use of mental health services: A population-based study in Ontario, 2002–2014. *Canadian Medical Association Journal, 192,* E329–E337.

Chivers-Wilson, K. (2006). Sexual assault and posttraumatic stress disorder: A review of the biological, psychological and sociological factors and treatments. *McGill Medical Journal, 9,* 111–118.

Cicchetti, D. (2010). Resilience under conditions of extreme stress: A multilevel perspective. *World Psychiatry, 9,* 145–154.

Cloitre, M., Garvert, D. W., Weiss, B., Carlson, E. B., & Bryan, R. A. (2014). Distinguishing PTSD, complex PTSD, and borderline personality disorder: A latent class analysis. *European Journal of Psychotraumatology, 5,* 25097.

Cohen, J. (1994): The earth is round (p<.05). *American Psychologist, 49,* 997–1003.

Cohen, J. R., Menon, S. V., Shorey, R. C., Le, V. D., & Temple, J. R. (2017). The distal consequences of physical and emotional neglect in emerging adults: A person-centered, multi-wave, longitudinal study. *Child Abuse & Neglect, 63,* 151–161.

Costa, P. T., & Widiger, T. A. (Eds.). (2015). *Personality disorders and the Five Factor Model of personality* (3rd ed.). American Psychological Association.

Coyne, S. M., Rogers, A. A., Zurcher, J. D., Stockdale, L., & Booth, M. (2019). Does time spent using social media impact mental health? An eight-year longitudinal study. *Faculty Publications,* 4124–4128.

Crowell, S., Beauchaine, T. P., & Linehan, M. M. (2009). A biosocial developmental model of borderline personality: elaborating and extending Linehan's theory. *Psychological Bulletin, 135,* 495–510.

Cuijpers, P., van Veen, S. C., Sijbrandij, M., Yoder, W., & Cristea, I. A. (2020). Eye movement desensitization and reprocessing for mental health problems: A systematic review and meta-analysis. *Cognitive Behaviour Therapy, 49*(3), 165–180.

Daskalakis, N. P., Rijal, C. M., King, C., Huckins, L. M., & Ressler, K. J. (2018). Recent genetics and epigenetics approaches to PTSD. *Current Psychiatry Reports, 20,* 30–41.

Deblinger, E., Mannarino, A. P., Cohen, J. A., & Steer, R. A. (2006). A follow-up study of a multisite, randomized, controlled trial for children with sexual abuse-related PTSD symptoms. *Journal of the American Academy of Child & Adolescent Psychiatry, 45,* 1474–1484.

Dennett, D. (2003). *Freedom evolves.* Penguin Random House.

DiGangi, J. A., Gomez, D., Mendoza, L., Jason, L. A., Keys, C. B., & Koenen, K. C. (2013). Pretrauma risk factors for posttraumatic stress disorder: A systematic review of the literature. *Clinical Psychology Review, 33,* 728–744.

Dohrenwend, B. P., Turner, J. B., Turse, N. A., Adams, B. G., Koenen, K. C., & Marshall, R. (2006). The psychological risks of Vietnam for U.S. veterans: A revisit with new data and methods. *Science, 313,* 979–982.

Dohrenwend, B. P., Turse, N. A., Yager, T. J., & Wall, M. M. (2019). *Surviving Vietnam: Psychological consequences of the war for US veterans.* Oxford University Press.

Dovran, A., Winje, D., Øverland, S., Arefjord, K., Hansen, A., & Waage, L. (2015). Childhood maltreatment and adult mental health. *Nordic Journal of Psychiatry, 70,* 140–145.

Duckers, E. A., & Brewin, C. B. (2016). A vulnerability paradox in the cross-national prevalence of post-traumatic stress disorder. *British Journal of Psychiatry, 209,* 300–305.

Duffy, M. E., Twenge, J. M., & Joiner, T. E. (2019). Trends in mood and anxiety symptoms and suicide-related outcomes among U.S. undergraduates, 2007–2018: Evidence from two national surveys. *Journal of Adolescent Psychology, 65,* 590–598.

Duncan, L. E., Raranatharathorn, A., Aiello, A. E., Almli, L. M., & Koenem, K. C. (2018). Largest GWAS of PTSD (N=20070) yields genetic overlap with schizophrenia and sex differences in heritability. *Molecular Psychiatry, 23,* 66–673.

Dunlop, B. W., & Wong, A., (2019). The hypothalamic-pituitary-adrenal axis in PTSD: Pathophysiology and treatment interventions. *Progress in Neuro-Psychopharmacology and Biological Psychiatry, 89,* 361–379.

Eaton, W. W., Sigal, J. J., & Weinfeld, M. (1982). Impairment in Holocaust survivors after 33 years: Data from an unbiased community sample. *American Journal of Psychiatry, 139,* 773–777.

Ehlers, A., Bisson, J., Clark, D. M., Creamer, M., Pilling, S., Richards, A., Schnurr, P. P., Turner, S., & Yule, W. (2010). Do all psychological treatments really work the same in posttraumatic stress disorder? *Clinical Psychology Review, 30,* 269–276.

Ehlers, A., & Clark, D. M. (2003). Early psychological interventions for adult survivors of trauma: A review. *Biological Psychiatry, 53,* 817–826.

Engel, G. L. (1980). The clinical application of the biopsychosocial model. *American Journal of Psychiatry, 137,* 535–544.

Engelhard, I., McNally, R. J., & van Schie, K. (2019). Retrieving and modifying traumatic memories: Recent research relevant to three controversies. *Current Directions in Psychological Science, 28,* 91–96.

Engelhard, I. M., van den Hout, M., & Kindt, M. (2003). The relationship between neuroticism, pre-traumatic stress, and post-traumatic stress: A prospective study. *Personality & Individual Differences, 35,* 381–388.

Everly, G., & Lating, J. (2019). *Clinical guide to the treatment of the human stress response* (4th ed.). Springer.

Farrington, D. P., Gallagher, B., Morley, L., St Ledger, R. J., & West, D. J. (1988). A 24-year follow-up of men from vulnerable backgrounds. In R. L. Jenkins & W. K. Brown (Eds.), *The abandonment of delinquent behaviour: Promoting the turnaround* (pp. 155–173). Praeger.

Fergusson, D., Boden, J., & Horwood, L. (2008). Exposure to childhood sexual and physical abuse and adjustment in early adulthood. *Child Abuse & Neglect, 32,* 607–619.

Fergusson, D. M., Horwood, L. J., & Lynskey, M. T. (1996a). Childhood sexual abuse and psychiatric disorder in young adulthood: II. Psychiatric outcomes of childhood sexual abuse. *Journal of the American Academy of Child & Adolescent Psychiatry, 35,* 1365–1374.

Fergusson, D. M., Horwood, L. J., Miller, A. L., & Kennedy, M. A. (2011). Life stress, 5-HTTLPR and mental disorder: Findings from a 30-year longitudinal study. *British Journal of Psychiatry, 198,* 129–135.

Fergusson, D. M., Lynskey, M. T., & Horwood, L. J. (1996b). Childhood sexual abuse and psychiatric disorder in young adulthood: I. Prevalence of sexual abuse and factors associated with sexual abuse. *Journal of the American Academy of Child & Adolescent Psychiatry, 35,* 1355–1364.

Fergusson, D., & Mullen, P. (1999). *Childhood sexual abuse: An evidence-based perspective.* Sage.

Finkelhor, D. (1990). Early and long-term effects of child sexual abuse: An update. *Professional Psychology: Research and Practice, 21,* 325–330.

Finkelhor, D., & Jones, L. M. (2006). Why have child maltreatment and child victimization declined? *Journal of Social Issues, 62,* 685–716.

Fisher, H., Caspi, A., & Arsenault, L. (2015). Measuring adolescents' exposure to victimization: The Environmental Risk (E-Risk) Longitudinal Twin Study. *Developmental Psychopathology, 27,* 1399–1416.

Flory, J. D., & Yehuda, R. (2015). Comorbidity between post-traumatic stress disorder and major depressive disorder: Alternative explanations and treatment considerations. *Dialogues in Clinical Neuroscience, 17,* 141–150.

Foa, E. B., & Kozak, M. J. (1986). Emotional processing of fear: Exposure to corrective information. *Psychological Bulletin, 99,* 20–35.

Foa, E. B., & Meadows, E. A. (1997). Psychosocial treatments for posttraumatic stress disorder: A critical review. *Annual Review of Psychology, 48,* 449–480.

Foa, E. B., Steketee, G., & Rothbaum, B. O. (1989). Behavioral/cognitive conceptualizations of post-traumatic stress disorder. *Behavior Therapy, 20,* 155–176.

Ford, J. D. (2020). New findings questioning the construct validity of complex posttraumatic stress disorder (cPTSD): Let's take a closer look. *European Journal of Psychotraumatology, 11,* article 1708145. https://doi.org/10.1080/20008198.2019.1708145

Ford, J. D., & Courtois, C. A. (2014). Complex PTSD, affect dysregulation, and borderline personality disorder. *Borderline Personality Disorder & Emotion Dysregulation, 1*, 9–16.

Fossati, A., Madeddu, F., & Maffei, C. (1999). Borderline personality disorder and childhood sexual abuse: A meta-analytic study. *Journal of Personality Disorders, 13*, 268–280.

Frances, A. (2013). *Saving normal.* Morrow.

Frank, J. D., & Frank, J. B. (1991). *Persuasion and healing* (3rd ed.). Johns Hopkins Press.

Freud, S. (1896/1962). The aetiology of hysteria. In J. Strachey (Ed.), *The standard edition of the psychological works of Sigmund Freud* (III: 191–224). Hogarth Press.

Frewen, P., Brown, M., DePierro, J., D'Andrea, W., & Schore, A. (2015). Assessing the family dynamics of childhood maltreatment history with the Childhood Attachment and Relational Trauma Screen (CARTS). *European Journal of Psychotraumatology, 6*, 27792.

Frost, R., Hyland, P., Shevlin, M., & Murphy, J. (2018). Distinguishing complex PTSD from borderline personality disorder among individuals with a history of sexual trauma: A latent class analysis. *European Journal of Trauma & Dissociation, 4*, 10.1016.

Frueh, B. C., Grubaugh, A. L., Madan, A., Neer, S. M., Elhai, J. D., & Beidel, D. C. (2018). Evidence-based practice for posttraumatic stress disorder. In D. David, S. J. Lynn, & G. H. Montgomery (Eds.), *Evidence-based psychotherapy: The state of the science and practice* (pp. 157–188). Wiley.

Furedi, F. (2004). *Therapy culture: Cultivating vulnerability in an uncertain age.* Routledge.

Ghaemi, N. (2010). *The rise and fall of the biopsychosocial model: Reconciling art and science in psychiatry.* Johns Hopkins University Press.

Gil, D. (2013). *Violence against children.* Harvard University Press.

Gilbert, D. T., Pinel, E. C., Wilson, T. D., Blumberg, S. J., & Wheatley, T. P. (1998). Immune neglect: A source of durability bias in affective forecasting. *Journal of Personality and Social Psychology, 75*, 617–638.

Gilbertson, M. W., Shenton, M. E., Ciszewski, A., Kasai, K., Lasko, N. B., Orr, S. P., & Pitman, R. K. (2002). Smaller hippocampal volume predicts pathologic vulnerability to psychological trauma. *Nature Neuroscience, 5*, 1242–1247.

Glueck, S., & Glueck, E. (1950). *Unraveling juvenile delinquency.* W. B. Saunders.

Goldberg, D., & Goodyer, I. (2005). *The origins and course of common mental disorders.* Taylor and Francis.

Gray, J. (2013). *The silence of animals: On progress and other modern myths.* Farrar, Strauss & Giroux.

Grob, G. N., & Horwitz, A. (2010). *Diagnosis, therapy, and evidence: Conundrums in modern American medicine.* Rutgers University Press.

Gross, J. J. (Ed.). (2014). *Handbook of emotion regulation.* Guilford.

Gunderson, J. G., & Sabo, A. N. (1993). The phenomenological and conceptual interface between borderline personality disorder and PTSD. *American Journal of Psychiatry, 150*, 19–27.

Haidt, J. (2012). *The righteous mind: Why good people are divided by politics and religion.* Pantheon.

Hailes, H., Yu, R., Danese, A., & Fazel, S. (2019). Long-term outcomes of childhood sexual abuse: An umbrella review. *Lancet Psychiatry, 6*(10), 830–839.

Harris, J. R. (1998). *The nurture assumption: Why children turn out the way they do.* Free Press.

Haslam, N. (2016). Concept creep: Psychology's expanding concepts of harm and pathology. *Psychological Inquiry, 27*, 1–17.

Hayes, S. (2012). *Acceptance and commitment therapy* (2nd ed.). Guilford.

Hayes, S., & Hoffman, S. G. (2017). The third wave of cognitive behavioral therapy and the rise of process-based care. *World Psychiatry, 16*, 245–254.

Henrich, J. (2020). *The WEIRDest people in the world: How the West became psychologically peculiar and particularly prosperous.* Farrar, Strauss & Giroux.

Herman, J. (1992). *Trauma and recovery.* Basic Books.

Hetrick, S. E., Purcell, R., Garner, B., & Parslow, R. (2010). Combined pharmacotherapy and psychological therapies for post-traumatic stress disorder (PTSD). *Cochrane Database of Systematic Reviews, 7*, CD007316.

Hevey, D. (2018). Network analysis: A brief overview and tutorial. *Health Psychology & Behavioral Medicine, 6*, 301–328.

Hinton, D. E., & Good, B. J. (Eds.). (2015). *Culture and PTSD: Trauma in global and historical perspective.* University of Pennsylvania Press.

Hinton, D. E., & Lewis-Fernandez, R. (2011). The cross-cultural validity of posttraumatic stress disorder: Implications for DSM-5. *Depression & Anxiety, 28*, 783–801.

Horwitz, A. V. (2018). *PTSD: A short history.* Johns Hopkins Press.

Hyer, L., Braswell, L., Albrecht, B., Boyd, S., Boudewyns, P., & Talbert, S. (1994). Relationship of NEO-PI to personality styles and severity of trauma in chronic PTSD victims. *Journal of Clinical Psychology, 50*, 699–707.

Institute of Medicine and National Research Council. (2014). *New directions in child abuse and neglect research.* National Academies Press. https://doi.org/10.17226/18331

Ioannidis, J. (2005). Why most published research findings are false. *PLOS Medicine, 2*(8), e124.

Janet, P. (1907). *The major symptoms of hysteria.* MacMillan.

Jang, K., Paris, J., Zweig-Frank, H., & Livesley, J. (1998). A twin study of dissociative experience. *Journal of Nervous and Mental Disease, 186*, 345–351.

Jang, K., Stein, M. B., Tayor, S., & Livesley, W. J. (2003). Exposure to traumatic events and experiences: Aetiological relationships with personality function. *Psychiatric Research, 120*, 61–69.

Johnson, J. G., Smailes, R. E. M., Cohen, P., Brown, J., & Bernstein, D. P. (2000). Associations between four types of childhood neglect and personality disorder symptoms during adolescence and early adulthood: Findings of a community-based longitudinal study. *Journal of Personality Disorders, 14*, 171–187.

Jones, E., Hodgins-Vermaas, R., McCartney, H., & Wessely, S. (2002). Post-combat syndromes from the Boer war to the Gulf war: A cluster analysis of their nature and attribution. *British Medical Journal, 324*, 321–324.

Jones, E., & Wessely, S. (2005). *Shell shock to PTSD: Military psychiatry from 1900 to the Gulf War.* Psychology Press.

Jones, P. J., Bellet, B., & McNally, R. J. (2020). Helping or harming? The effect of trigger warnings on individuals with trauma histories. *Clinical Psychological Science, 29*, 1–13.

Kagan, J. (1994). *Galen's prophecy.* Basic Books.

Kagan, J. (1998). *Three seductive ideas.* Harvard University Press.

Kahnemann, D. (2011). *Thinking fast and slow.* Farrar, Strauss and Giroux.

Kaminer, W. (1992). *I'm dysfunctional, you're dysfunctional: The recovery movement and other self-help fashions.* Addison-Wesley.

Kar, N. (2011). Cognitive behavioral therapy for the treatment of post-traumatic stress disorder: A review. *Neuropsychiatric Disease & Treatment, 7*, 167–181.

Karatzias, T., Shevlin, M., Fyvie, C., Hyland, P., Efthymiadou, E., Wilson, D., Roberts, N., Bisson, J. I., Brewin, C. R., & Cloitre, M. (2017). Evidence of distinct profiles of posttraumatic stress disorder (PTSD) and complex posttraumatic stress disorder (CPTSD) based on the new ICD-11 Trauma Questionnaire (ICD-T). *Journal of Affective Disorders, 207*, 181–187.

Katerndahl, D., Burge, S., & Kellogg, N. (2005). Predictors of development of adult psychopathology in female victims of childhood sexual abuse. *Journal of Nervous and Mental Disease, 193*, 258–264.

Kendler, K., & Prescott, C. (2007). *Genes, environment and psychopathology.* Guilford.

Kessler, R. C., Aguilar-Gaxiola, S., Alonso, J., Benjet, C., Bromet, E. J., Cardoso, G., Degenhardt, L., de Girolamo, G., Dinolova, R. V., Ferry, F., Florescu, S., Gureje, O., Haro, J. M., Huang, Y., Karam, E. G., Kawakami, N., Lee, S., Lepine, J-P., Levinson, D., . . . Koenen, K. C. (2017). Trauma and PTSD in the WHO World Mental Health Surveys. *European Journal of Psychotraumatology, 8*(Suppl. 5), 1353383.

Kessler, R. C., Avenovli, S., Costello, J., Georgiades, K., Green, J. G., Gruber, M. J., He, J., Koretz, D., McLaughlin, K. A., Petukhova, M., Sampson, N. A., Zaslavsky, A. M., & Merkangas, K. R. (2012). Prevalence, persistence, and sociodemographic correlates of DSM-IV disorders in the National Comorbidity Survey Replication Adolescent Supplement. *Archives of General Psychiatry, 69*, 372–380.

Kessler, R. C., Berglund, P., Demler, O., Jin, R., & Walters, E. E. (2005a). Lifetime prevalence and age-of-onset distributions of DSM-IV disorders in the National Comorbidity Survey Replication. *Archives of General Psychiatry, 62*, 593–602.

Kessler, R. C., Demler, O., & Frank, R. G. (2005b). Prevalence and treatment of mental disorders, 1990 to 2003. *New England Journal of Medicine, 352,* 2515–2523.

Kessler, R. C., Sonnega, A., Bromet, E., Hughes, M., & Nelson, C. B. (1995). Posttraumatic stress disorder in the National Comorbidity Survey. *Archives of General Psychiatry, 52,* 1048–1060.

Kihlstrom, J. F. (1987). The cognitive unconscious. *Science, 18*(237), 1445–1452.

Kilpatrick, D., Resnick, H., Milanak, M., Miller, M., Keyes, K. M., & Friedman, M. J. (2013). National estimates of exposure to traumatic events and PTSD prevalence using DSM-IV and DSM-5 criteria. *Journal of Traumatic Stress, 26,* 537–547.

Kirmayer, L. J., Barad, M., & Lemelson, R. (Eds.). (2007). *Understanding trauma: Integrating biological, clinical, and cultural perspectives.* Cambridge University Press.

Knopik, B., Neiderheise, J. M., DeFries, J. C., & Plomin, R. (2017). *Behavioral genetics* (7th ed.). Worth.

Knowles, K. A., Sripada, R. K., Defever, M., & Rauch, S. A. M. (2019). Comorbid mood and anxiety disorders and severity of posttraumatic stress disorder symptoms in treatment-seeking veterans. *Psychological Trauma, 11,* 451–458.

Knox, J. (2011). *Self-agency in psychotherapy: Attachment, autonomy, and intimacy.* Norton.

Koenen, K. C., Nugent, N. R., & Amstadter, S. M. (2008). Gene–environment interaction in posttraumatic stress disorder: Review, strategy and new directions for future research. *European Archives of Psychiatry & Clinical Neuroscience, 258,* 82–96.

Kotov, R., Krueger, R. F., Watson, D., Achenbach, T. M., Althoff, R. R., Bagby, R. M., Brown, T. A., Carpenter, W. T., Caspi, A., Clark, L. A., Eaton, N. R., Forbes, M. K., Forbush, K. T., Goldberg, D., Hasin, D., Hyman, S. E., Ivanova, M. Y., Lynam, D. R., Markon, K., . . . Zimmerman, M. (2017). The Hierarchical Taxonomy of Psychopathology (HiTOP): A dimensional alternative to traditional nosologies. *Journal of Abnormal Psychology, 126,* 454–477.

Kraemer, H. C., Stice, E. C., Kazdin, A., Offord, D., & Kupfer, D. (2001). How do risk factors work together? Mediators, moderators, and independent, overlapping, and proxy risk factors. *American Journal of Psychiatry, 158,* 848–856.

Kramer, E. J., Kwong, K., & Chung, E. (2002). Cultural factors influencing the mental health of Asian Americans. *Western Medicine, 176,* 226–231.

Kulka, R. A., Schlenger, W. E., Fairbank, J., & Hough, R. L. (1990). *Trauma and the Vietnam War generation.* Brunner/Mazel.

Lancaster, C. L., Teeters, J. B., Gros, D. F., & Back, S. E. (2016). Posttraumatic stress disorder: Overview of evidence-based assessment and treatment. *Journal of Clinical Medicine, 5,* 105–117.

Lanius, R., & Olff, M. (2017). The neurobiology of PTSD. *European Journal of Psychotraumatology, 8,* 1314165.

Laporte, L., Paris, J., Russell, J., Guttman, H., & Correa, J. (2012). Childhood trauma in patients with borderline personality disorder and their sisters. *Child Maltreatment, 17*, 318–329.

Laporte, L., Paris, J., Zelkowitz, P., & Cardin, J. F. (2018). Clinical outcomes of a stepped care program for the treatment of borderline personality disorder. *Personality and Mental Health, 12*, 252–264.

Lee, W., Lee, Y. R., Yoon, J. H., Lee, H. J., & Kang, M. Y. (2020). Occupational post-traumatic stress disorder: An updated systematic review. *BMC Public Health, 20*, 768. https://doi.org/10.1186/s12889-020-08903-2

Leenarts, L., Diehl, J., Jansma, E. P., & Lindauer, R. (2013). Evidence-based treatments for children with trauma-related psychopathology as a result of childhood maltreatment: A systematic review. *European Child and Adolescent Psychiatry, 22*, 269–283.

Lehrner, A., & Yehuda, R. (2020). PTSD diagnoses and treatments: Closing the gap between ICD-11 and DSM-5. *BJPsych Advances, 26*, 153–155.

Leighton, D. C., Harding, J. S., & Macklin, D. B. (1963). *The character of danger: Psychiatric symptoms in selected communities.* Basic Books.

Lewis, M. (1997). *Altering fate.* Guilford.

Lewis, S., Caspi, A., Arsenault, L., Fisher, H. L., Matthews, T., Moffitt, T. E., Odgers, C. L., Stahl, D., Teng, J. Y., & Danese, A. (2019). The epidemiology of trauma and post-traumatic stress disorder in a representative cohort of young people in England and Wales. *Lancet Psychiatry, 6*, 247–256.

Lichtenstein, P., Yip, B. H., Bjork, C., & Pawitan, Y. (2009). Common genetic determinants of schizophrenia and bipolar disorder in Swedish families: A population-based study. *Lancet, 373*(9659), 234–239.

Linehan, M. M. (1993). *Cognitive behavior therapy for borderline personality disorder.* Guilford.

Lippard, E., & Nemeroff, C. (2020). The devastating clinical consequences of child abuse and neglect: Increased disease vulnerability and poor treatment response in mood disorders. *American Journal of Psychiatry, 177*, 20–36.

Liu, R. T. (2019). Childhood maltreatment and impulsivity: A meta-analysis and recommendations for future study. *Journal of Abnormal Child Psychology, 47*, 221–243.

Livesley, W. J., Jang, K. L., & Vernon, P. A. (1998). Phenotypic and genetic structure of traits delineating personality disorder. *Archives of General Psychiatry, 55*, 941–948.

Loftus, E. F., & Ketcham, K. (1994). *The myth of repressed memory.* St. Martin's Press.

Lohr, J. M., Gist, R., Deacon, B., Devilly, G. J., & Varker, T. (2014). Science- and non-science-based treatments for trauma-related stress disorders. In S. Lilienfeld, S. J. Lynn, & J. Lohr (Eds.), *Science and pseudoscience in clinical psychology.* Guilford.

Loring, M. T. (1994). *Emotional abuse.* Lexington Books/Macmillan.

Lowell, A., Suarez-Jimenez, B., Helpman, L., Zhu, X., Durosky, A., Hilburn, A., Schneier, F., Gross, R., & Neria, Y. (2018). 9/11-related PTSD among highly exposed populations: A systematic review 15 years after the attack. *Psychological Medicine, 48*, 537–553.

Lukianoff, G., & Haidt, J. (2018). *The coddling of the American mind: How good intentions and bad ideas are setting up a generation for failure.* Penguin Publishing Group.

Lykken, D. (1995). *The antisocial personalities.* Lawrence Erlbaum.

Lynn, S. J., Evans, J., Laurence, J. R., & Lilienfeld, S. O. (2015). What do people believe about memory? Implications for the science and pseudoscience of clinical practice. *Canadian Journal of Psychiatry, 60*, 541–547.

Lyons, M. J., Goldberg, J., Eisen, S. A., True, W., Meyer, J., Tsuang, M. T., & Henderson, W. (1993). Do genes influence exposure to trauma? A twin study of combat. *American Journal of Medical Genetics, 48*, 22–27.

Maercker, A., Mohiyeddini, C., Müller, M., Xie, W., Hui Yang, Z., Wang, J., & Müller, J. (2011). Traditional versus modern values, self-perceived interpersonal factors, and posttraumatic stress in Chinese and German crime victims. *Journal of Child Psychology and Psychiatry, 82*, 219–232.

Maguen, S., Metzler, T. J., McCaslin, S. E., Inslicht, S. S., Henn-Haase, C., Neylan, T. C., & Marmar, C. R. (2009). Routine work environment stress and PTSD symptoms in police officers. *Journal of Nervous and Mental Disease, 197*, 754–760.

Markham, M., Lutz, W., & Castongauy, L. (2021). *Bergin and Garfield's Handbook of Psychotherapy and Behavior Change,* 7th Edition. New York: John Wiley.

Markowitz, J. C., Petkova, E., Neria, Y., van Meter, P. E., Zhao, Y., Hembree, E., Lovell, E., Biyanova, T., & Marshall, R. D. (2015). Is exposure necessary? A randomized clinical trial of interpersonal psychotherapy for PTSD. *American Journal of Psychiatry, 132*, 430–440.

Markus, H. R., & Kitayama, S. (1991). Culture and the self: Implications for cognition, emotion, and motivation. *Psychological Review, 98*, 224–253.

Marmar, C. R., Schlenger, W., Henn-Hasse, C., & Qian, M. (2015). Course of posttraumatic stress disorder 40 years after the Vietnam War: Findings from the National Vietnam Veterans Longitudinal Study. *JAMA Psychiatry, 72*, 875–881.

Mattson, E., James, L., & Engdahl, B. (2018). Personality factors and their impact on PTSD and post-traumatic growth is mediated by coping style among OIF/OEF veterans. *Military Medicine, 183*, 475–480.

McCauley, J., Killeen, T., Gros, D. F., Bradyn, K. T. et al. (2012). Posttraumatic Stress Disorder and Co-Occurring Substance Use Disorders: Advances in Assessment and Treatment. *Clin Psychol Sci Practice 19*, 293–304.

McCord, J. (1983). A forty-year perspective on effects of child abuse and neglect. *Child Abuse Negl;7*, 265–270.

McFarlane, A. C. (1988). The aetiology of post-traumatic stress disorders following a natural disaster. *British Journal of Psychiatry, 152*, 116–121.

McHugh, P. R. (2008). *Try to remember: Psychiatry's clash over meaning, memory, and mind.* Dana Press.

McNally, R. J. (1999). EMDR and mesmerism: A comparative historical analysis. *Journal of Anxiety Disorders, 13,* 225–236.

McNally, R. J. (2003). *Remembering trauma.* Harvard University Press.

McNally, R. J. (2006). Let Freud rest in peace. *Brain & Behavioral Sciences, 29,* 526–527.

McNally, R. J. (2007). Mechanisms of exposure therapy: How neuroscience can improve psychological treatments for anxiety disorders. *Clinical Psychology Review, 7,* 750–759.

McNally, R. J. (2012). The ontology of posttraumatic stress disorder: Natural kind, social construction, or causal system? *Clinical Psychology: Science and Practice, 19,* 220–228.

McNally, R. J. (2015). Is PTSD a transhistorical phenomenon? In D. E. Hinton & B. J. Good (Eds.), *Culture and PTSD: Trauma in global and historical perspective* (pp. 117–133). University of Pennsylvania Press.

McNally, R. J. (2016). The expanding empire of psychopathology: The case of PTSD. *Psychological Inquiry, 27*(1), 46–49.

McNally, R. J. (2017). Networks and nosology in posttraumatic stress disorder. *JAMA Psychiatry, 74,* 124–125.

McNally, R. J. (2018). Resolving the vulnerability paradox in the cross-national prevalence of posttraumatic stress disorder. *Journal of Anxiety Disorders, 54,* 33–35.McNally, R., Bryant, R. A., & Ehlers, A. (2003). Does early psychological intervention promote recovery from posttraumatic stress? *Psychological Science in the Public Interest, 4,* 45–79.

McNally, R. J., & Frueh, B. C. (2013). Why are Iraq and Afghanistan War veterans seeking PTSD disability compensation at unprecedented rates? *Journal of Anxiety Disorders, 27,* 520–526.

McNally, R. J., Heeren, A., & Robinaugh, D. J. (2017). A Bayesian network analysis of posttraumatic stress disorder symptoms in adults reporting childhood sexual abuse. *European Journal of Psychotraumatology, 8*(Supp. 3), 1341276.

Miller, M. W. (2003). Personality and the etiology and expression of PTSD: A three-factor model perspective. *Clinical Psychology: Science and Practice, 10,* 373–393.

Miller, M. W., Vogt, D. S., Mozley, S. L., Kaloupek, D. G., & Keane, T. M. (2006). PTSD and substance-related problems: The mediating roles of disconstraint and negative emotionality. *Journal of Abnormal Psychology, 115,* 369–379.

Millon, T., & Davis, R. (1995). *Personality disorders: DSM-IV and beyond.* Wiley.

Mitchell, J. T., & Everly, G. S., Jr. (2000). *Psychological debriefing: Theory, practice and evidence.* Cambridge University Press.

Monroe, S. M., & Harknessm, K. L., (2005). Life stress, the "kindling" hypothesis, and the recurrence of depression: Considerations from a life stress perspective. *Psychological Review, 112,* 417–445.

Mosing, M. A., Zietsch, B. P., Shekar, S. N., Wright, M. J., & Martin, N. G. (2009). Genetic and environmental influences on optimism and its relationship to mental and self-rated health: A study of aging twins. *Behavior Genetics, 39*, 597–604.

Mulder, R. T., Beautrais, A., Joyce, P. R., & Fergusson, D. (1998). Relationship between dissociation, childhood sexual abuse, childhood physical abuse, and mental illness in a general population sample. *American Journal of Psychiatry, 155*, 806–811.

Muldoon, O. T., Haslam, S. A., Haslam, C., Cruwys, T., Kearns, M., & Jetten, J. (2019). The social psychology of responses to trauma: Social identity pathways associated with divergent traumatic responses. *European Review of Social Psychology, 30*, 311–348.

Nash, M. R., Hulsey, T. L., Sexton, M. C., Harralson, T. L., & Lambert, W. (1993). Long-term sequelae of childhood sexual abuse: Perceived family environment, psychopathology, and dissociation. *Journal of Consulting and Clinical Psychology, 61*, 276–283.

Nathan, D. (2011). *Sibyl exposed.* Simon and Schuster.

National Institute for Clinical Excellence. (2018). *Post-traumatic stress disorder.* NICE Guidelines. www.nice.org.uk/guidance/ng116

Nesse, R. (2019). *Good reasons for bad feelings.* Oxford University Press.

Newbury, J. B., Arseneault, L., Moffitt, T. E., Caspi, A., Danese, A., Baldwin, J. R., & Fisher, H. L. (2018). Measuring childhood maltreatment to predict early adult psychopathology: Comparison of prospective informant-reports and retrospective self-reports. *Journal of Psychiatric Research, 96*, 57–64.

Nievergelt, C. M., Maihofer, A. X., Klengel, T., Atkinson, E. G., Chen, C-Y., Choi, K. W., Coleman, J. R. I., Dalvie, S., Duncan, L. E., Gelernter, J., Levey, D. F., Logue, M. W., Polimanti, R., Provost, A. C., Ratanatharathorn, A., Stein, M. B., Torres, K., Aiello, A. E., Almli, L. M., . . . Koenen, K. C. (2019). International meta-analysis of PTSD genome-wide association studies identifies sex- and ancestry-specific genetic risk loci. *Nature Communications, 10*, 4558.

Noll, J. G. (2021). Child sexual abuse as a unique risk factor for the development of psychopathology: The compounded convergence of mechanisms. *Annual Review of Clinical Psychology, 17*, 439–464. https://doi.org/10.1146/annurev-clinpsy-081219-112621

Norman, R. E., Byambaa, M., De, R., Butchart, A., Scott, J., & Vos. T. (2012). The long-term health consequences of child physical abuse, emotional abuse, and neglect: A systematic review and meta-analysis. *PloS Medicine, 9*(11), e1001349.

North, C. S., Suris, A. M., Davis, M., & Smith, R. P. (2009). Toward validation of the diagnosis of posttraumatic stress disorder. *American Journal of Psychiatry, 166*, 34–41.

O'Donnell, K., & Meaney, M. J. (2020). Epigenetics, development, and psychopathology. *Annual Review of Clinical Psychology, 16*, 10.1146.

Ogle, C. M., Rubin, D. C., Berntsen, D., & Siegler, I. C. (2013). The frequency and impact of exposure to potentially traumatic events over the life course. *Clinical Psychological Science, 1*(4), 426–434.

Olfson, M., Wang, S., Wall, M., Marcus, S. C., & Blanco, C. (2019). Trends in serious psychological distress and outpatient mental health care of US adults *JAMA Psychiatry, 76*, 152–161.

Ost, J., Easton, S., Hope, L., French, C. C., & Wright, D. B. (2017). Latent variables underlying the memory beliefs of chartered clinical psychologists, hypnotherapists and undergraduate students. *Memory, 25*, 57–68.

Otgaar, H., Howe, M. L., & Pathis, L. (2021). What science tells us about false and repressed memories. *Memory.* Advance online publication. https://doi.org/10.1080/09658211.2020.1870699

Otgaar, H., Loftus, E., Howe, M., Wang, J., Lynn, S. J., Merckelbach, H., & Patihis, L. (2020). Belief in unconscious repressed memory is widespread: A comment on Brewin, Li, Ntarantana, Unsworth, and McNeilis. *Journal of Experimental Psychology: General, 149*(10), 1996–2000.

Ozbay, F., Johnson, D. V., & Southwick, S. (2007). Social support and resilience to stress. *Psychiatry, 4*, 35–40.

Pagura, J., Bolton, J. M., Stein, M. B., & Cox, B. J. (2010). Comorbidity of borderline personality disorder and posttraumatic stress disorder in the U.S. population. *Journal of Psychiatric Research, 44*, 1190–1198.

Paris, J. (2000a). Predispositions, personality traits, and posttraumatic stress disorder. *Harvard Review of Psychiatry, 8*(4), 175–183.

Paris, J. (2000b). *Myths of childhood.* Brunner/Mazel.

Paris, J. (2012). The rise and fall of dissociative disorders. *Journal of Nervous and Mental Disease, 200*, 1076–1079.

Paris, J. (2013a). *Fads and fallacies in psychiatry.* Royal College of Psychiatrists.

Paris, J. (2013b). *Psychotherapy in an age of narcissism.* Palgrave Macmillan.

Paris, J. (2017). *Stepped care for borderline personality disorder: Making treatment brief, effective, and accessible.* Academic Press (Elsevier).

Paris, J. (2019). *An evidence-based critique of contemporary psychoanalysis.* Routledge.

Paris, J. (2020a). *Treatment of borderline personality disorder: A guide to evidence-based practice* (2nd ed., revised and updated). Guilford Press.

Paris, J. (2020b). *Social factors in the personality disorders* (2nd ed.). Cambridge University Press.

Paris, J. (2020c). *Overdiagnosis in psychiatry* (2nd ed.). Oxford University Press.

Paris, J. (2020d). *Nature and nurture in psychiatry: A gene–environment model* (2nd ed., revised and updated). American Psychiatric Publishing.

Paris, J. (2022). *Nature and Nurture in Personality and Psychopathology: A Guide for Clinicians.* London, UK: Routledge.

Paris, J., Zweig-Frank, H., & Guzder, J. (1994a). Psychological risk factors for borderline personality disorder in female patients. *Comprehensive Psychiatry, 35*, 301–305.

Paris, J., Zweig-Frank, H., & Guzder, J. (1994b). Risk factors for borderline personality in male outpatients. *Journal of Nervous and Mental Disease, 182,* 375–380.

Patten, S. B., Wang, J. L., Williams, J. V. A., Currie, S., Beck, C. A., Maxwell, C. J., & El-Guebaly, N. (2006). Descriptive epidemiology of major depression in Canada. *Canadian Journal of Psychiatry, 51,* 84–90.

Pineles, S. L., Hall, K., & Rasmusson, A. (2017). Gender and PTSD: Different pathways to a similar phenotype. *Current Opinion in Psychology, 14,* 44–48.

Pinker, S. (2012). *The better angels of our nature.* Penguin.

Pinker, S. (2019). *Enlightenment now.* Penguin.

Piper, A., Lillevik, L., & Kritzer, R. (2008). What's wrong with believing in repression? A review for legal professionals. *Psychology, Public Policy, and Law, 14,* 223–242.

Pitman, R. K., Gilbertson, M. W., Gurvits, T. V., May, F. S., Lasko, N. B., Metzger, L. J., Shenton, M. E., Yehuda, R., & Orr, S. P. (2006). Clarifying the origin of biological abnormalities in PTSD through the study of identical twins discordant for combat exposure. *Annals of the New York Academy of Science, 1071,* 242–254.

Plomin, R. (2018). *Blueprint: How DNA makes us who we are.* MIT Press.

Plomin, R., DeFries, J. C., Knopik, V. S., & Neiderhiser, J. M. (2016). Top 10 replicated findings from behavioral genetics. *Perspectives in Psychological Science, 11,* 3–23.

Porter, C., Palmier-Claus, J. M., Branitsky, A., Mansell, W., Warwick, H., & Varese, F. (2020). Childhood adversity and borderline personality disorder: A meta-analysis. *Acta Psychiatrica Scandinavica, 141,* 6–20.

Poulton, R., Moffitt, T. E., & Silva, P. A. (2015). The Dunedin Multidisciplinary Health and Development Study: Overview of the first 40 years, with an eye to the future. *Social Psychiatry, Psychiatry, and Epidemiology, 50,* 679–693.

Rauch, S., Eftekhari, K., & Ruzek, J. L. (2012). Review of exposure therapy: A gold standard? *Journal of Rehabilitation Research and Development, 49,* 679–688.

Rauch, S., & Foa, E. (2006). Emotional processing theory (EPT) and exposure therapy for PTSD. *Journal of Contemporary Psychotherapy, 36,* 61–65.

Read, J. D., & Lindsay, S. S. (1997). *Recollections of trauma: Scientific evidence and clinical practice.* Springer.

Regehr, C., & Marziali, E. (1999). Response to sexual assault: A relational perspective. *Journal of Nervous and Mental Disease, 187,* 618–623.

Resick, P. A., & Schnicke, P. A. (1993). *Cognitive processing therapy for rape victims: A treatment manual.* Sage.

Rind, B., & Tromovitch, P. (1997). A meta-analytic review of findings from national samples on psychological correlates of child sexual abuse. *Journal of Sexual Research, 34,* 237–255.

Rind, B., Tromovitch, P., & Bauserman, R. (1998). A meta-analytic examination of assumed properties of child sexual abuse using college samples. *Psychological Bulletin, 124,* 22–53.

Robertson, D. G., & Codd, T. (2019). Stoic philosophy as a cognitive-behavioral therapy. *The Behavior Therapist, 42,* 42–50.

Robins, L. N. (1966). *Deviant Children Grown Up*. Baltimore, MD: Williams & Wilkins.

Robins, L. N., & Regier, D. A. (1991). *Psychiatric disorders in America*. Free Press.

Robinson, H. M., Sigman, M. R., & Wilson, J. P. (1997). Duty-related stressors and PTSD symptoms in suburban police officers. *Psychological Reports, 81*, 835–845.

Rowland, T., & Marwaha, S. (2018). Epidemiology and risk factors for bipolar disorder. *Therapeutic Advances in Psychopharmacology, 8*, 251–269.

Rutter, M. (2006). *Genes and behavior: Nature–nurture interplay explained*. Blackwell.

Rutter, M. (2013). Annual research review: Resilience—clinical implications. *Journal of Child Psychology and Psychiatry, 54*, 474–487.

Rutter, M., & Quinton, D. (1984). Long-term follow-up of women institutionalized in childhood. *British Journal of Developmental Psychology, 18*, 225–234.

Rutter, M., Kumsta, R., Schlotz, W., & Sonuga-Barle, E. (2012). Longitudinal studies using a "natural experiment" design: The case of adoptees from Romanian institutions. *Journal of the American Academy of Child and Adolescent Psychiatry, 51*, 762–770.

Rutter, M., O'Connor, T. G., & English and Romanian Adoptees (ERA) Study Team. (2004). Are there biological programming effects for psychological development? Findings from a study of Romanian adoptees. *Developmental Psychology, 40*, 81–94.

Rutter, M., & Rutter, M. (1993). *Developing minds: Challenge and continuity across the life span*. Basic Books.

Rutter, M., Tizard, J., Yule, W., Graham, P., & Whitmore, K. (1976). Isle of Wight studies, 1964–1974. *Psychological Medicine, 6*, 313–332.

Ryan, J., Chaudieu, I., Ancelin, M. L., & Saffery, R. (2016). Biological underpinnings of trauma and post-traumatic stress disorder: Focusing on genetics and epigenetics. *Epigenomics, 8*, 1553–1569.

Samuel, D. B., & Widiger, T. A. (2008). A meta-analytic review of the relationships between the five-factor model and DSM-IV-TR personality disorders: A facet-level analysis. *Clinical Psychology Review, 28*, 1326–1342.

Sareen, J. (2014). Post-traumatic stress disorder in adults: Impact, comorbidity risk factors and treatment. *Canadian Journal of Psychiatry, 59*, 460–467.

Sartor, C. E., Grant, J. D., Lynskey, M. T., & Nelson, E. C. (2012). Common heritable contributions to low-risk trauma, high-risk trauma, posttraumatic stress disorder, and major depression. *Archives of General Psychiatry, 69*, 293–299.

Satel, S., & Lilienfeld, S. O. (2013). *Brainwashed: The seductive appeal of mindless neuroscience*. Basic Books.

Schacter, D. L. (2001). *The seven sins of memory: How the mind forgets and remembers*. Houghton Mifflin.

Schacter, D. L. (2008). *Searching for memory*. Basic Books.

Scheeringa, M. S. (2008). Developmental considerations for diagnosing PTSD and acute stress disorder in preschool and school-age children. *American Journal of Psychiatry, 165*, 1237–1240.

Scheiderer, E. M., Wood, P. K., & Trull, T. J. (2015). The comorbidity of border-line personality disorder and posttraumatic stress disorder: Revisiting the prevalence and associations in a general population sample. *Borderline Personality Disorder and Emotion Dysregulation, 2*, 11–21.

Schlenger, W. E., Kulka, R. A., Fairbank, J. A., Hough, R. L., Marmar, C. R., & Weiss, D. S. (1992). The prevalence of post-traumatic stress disorder in the Vietnam generation: A multimethod, multisource assessment of psychiatric disorder. *Journal of Traumatic Stress, 5*, 333–363.

Schmitt, D. P., Realo, A., Voracek, M., & Alik, J. (2008). Why can't a man be more like a woman? Sex differences in Big Five personality traits across 55 cultures. *Journal of Personality and Social Psychology, 94*, 168–192.

Schreiber, F. R. (1973). *Sibyl*. Henry Regnery.

Schwartz, H. S. (1994). Beyond individualism/collectivism: New cultural dimensions of values. In U. Kim & H. Triandis (Eds.), *Individualism and collectivism: Theory, method and application* (pp. 85–119). Sage.

Scott, W. J. (1990). PTSD in DSM-III: A case in the politics of diagnosis and disease. *Social Problems, 37*, 294–310.

Seedat, S., & Stein, M. B. (2001). Post-traumatic stress disorder: A review of recent findings. *Current Psychiatric Reports, 3*, 288–294.

Segal, Z. V., Williams, M. G., & Teasdale, J. D. (Eds.). (2013). *Mindfulness-based cognitive therapy for depression* (2nd ed.). Guilford Press.

Seidler, G., & Wagner, F. (2013). Comparing the efficacy of EMDR and trauma-focused cognitive-behavioral therapy in the treatment of PTSD: A meta-analytic study. *Psychological Medicine, 36*, 515–521.

Shalev, A. Y., Peri, T., Brandes, D., Freedman, S., Orr, S. P., & Pitman, R. K. (2000). Auditory startle response in trauma survivors with posttraumatic stress disorder: A prospective study. *American Journal of Psychiatry, 157*, 255–261.

Shapiro, F. (1989). Efficacy of the eye movement desensitization procedure in the treatment of traumatic memories. *Journal of Traumatic Stress, 2*, 199–223.

Sheerin, C. M., Lind, M. J., Bountress, K., Nugent, N. R., & Amstadter, A. B. (2017). The genetics and epigenetics of PTSD: Overview, recent advances, and future directions. *Current Opinion in Psychology, 14*, 5–11.

Shermer, M. (2011). *The believing brain: From ghosts and gods to politics and conspiracies: How we construct beliefs and reinforce them as truths*. St. Martin's Griffin.

Shields, M., Tonmyr, L., & Hovdestad, W. (2016). Is child sexual abuse declining in Canada? Results from nationally representative retrospective surveys. *Health Promotion and Chronic Disease Prevention in Canada: Research, Policy and Practice, 36*, 252–260.

Shields, M., Tonmyr, L., & Hovdestad, W. E. (2019). The decline of child sexual abuse in Canada: Evidence from the 2014 General Social Survey. *Canadian Journal of Psychiatry, 64*, 638–646.

Shorter, E. (1997). *A history of psychiatry*. Free Press.

Sigal, J. J., & Weinfeld, M. (2001). Do children cope better than adults with potentially traumatic stress? A 40-year follow-up of Holocaust survivors. *Psychiatry: Interpersonal and Biological Processes, 64*, 69–78.

Snarey, J. R., & Vaillant, G. E. (1985). How lower- and working-class youth become middle-class adults: The association between ego defense mechanisms and upward social mobility. *Child Development, 56*, 899–910.

Soloff, P., & Chiappetta, L. (2019). 10-Year Outcome of suicidal behavior in borderline personality disorder. *Journal of Personality Disorders, 33*, 82–100.

Speer, K. R., Semple, S., Naumovski, N., D'Cunha, N. M., & McKune, A. J. (2019). HPA axis function and diurnal cortisol in post-traumatic stress disorder: A systematic review. *Neurobiology of Stress, 11*, 100180.

Stoltenborgh, M., Bakermans-Kranenburg, M. J., & van IJzendoorn, M. H. (2013). The neglect of child neglect: A meta-analytic review of the prevalence of neglect. *Social Psychiatry and Psychiatric Epidemiology, 48*, 345–355.

Southwick, S. M., & Charney, D. S. (2018). *Resilience: The science of mastering life's greatest challenges*. Cambridge University Press.

Stein, D. J., Zungu-Dirwayi, N., van der Linden, G. J., & Seedat, S. (2000). Pharmacotherapy for posttraumatic stress disorder. *Cochrane Database of Systematic Reviews, 4*, CD002795. doi:10.1002/14651858.CD002795

Stein, M. B., Jang, K. L., & Livesley, W. J. (1999). Heritability of anxiety sensitivity: A twin study. *American Journal of Psychiatry, 156*, 246–251.

Stein, M. B., Jang, K. L., Vernon, P. A., & Livesley, W. J. (2002). Genetic and environmental influences on trauma exposure and posttraumatic stress disorder symptoms: A twin study. *American Journal of Psychiatry, 159*, 1675–1681.

Summerfield, D. (2001). The invention of post-traumatic stress disorder and the social usefulness of a psychiatric category. *British Medical Journal, 322*, 95–98.

Taleb, N. N. (2012). *Antifragile: Things that gain from disorder*. Random House.

Tedeschi, R. J., Shakespeare-Finch, R., Taku, K., & Calhoun, L. G. (2018). *Posttraumatic growth: Theory, research, and applications*. Routledge.

Terr, L. C. (1988). What happens to early memories of trauma? *Journal of the American Academy of Child and Adolescent Psychiatry, 27*, 96–104.

Thigpen, C. H., & Cleckley, H. M. (1957). *The three faces of Eve* Houghton Mifflin.

Tolin, D. F., & Foa, E. B. (2006). Sex differences in trauma and posttraumatic stress disorder: A quantitative review of 25 years of research. *Psychological Bulletin, 132*, 959–992.

Tremblay, R., Vitaro, F., & Cote, S. M. (2018). Developmental origins of chronic physical aggression: A bio-psycho-social model for the next generation of preventive intervention. *Annual Review of Psychology, 69*, 383–407.

Trouton, A., Spinath, F. M., & Plomin, R. (2002). Twins Early Development Study (TEDS): A multivariate, longitudinal genetic investigation of language, cognition and behaviour problems in childhood. *Twin Research, 38*, 444–448.

True, W. R., Rice, J., Eisen, S. A., Heath, A. C., Goldberg, J., Lyons, M. J., & Nowak, J. (1993). A twin study of genetic and environmental contributions to liability for post-traumatic stress symptoms. *Archives of General Psychiatry, 50,* 257–264.

Twenge, J. M., Martin, G. N., & Campbell, W. K. (2018). Decreases in psychological well-being among American adolescents after 2012 and links to screen time during the rise of smartphone technology. *Emotion, 18,* 765–780.

Vaillant, G. E. (2012). *Triumphs of experience: The men of the Harvard Grant Study.* Harvard University Press.

Van der Kolk, B. A. (2014). *The body keeps the score: Brain, mind and body in the healing of trauma.* Penguin.

van Emmerik, A. A. P., Kamphuis, J. H., Hulsbosch, A. M., & Emmelkamp, P. (2002). Single session debriefing after psychological trauma: A meta-analysis. *Lancet, 360,* 766–771.

van Zuiden, M., Geuze, E., Willemen, H. L. D. M., Vermetten, E., Maas, M., Heijnen, C. J., & Kavelaars, A. (2011). Pre-existing high glucocorticoid receptor number predicting development of posttraumatic stress symptoms after military deployment. *American Journal of Psychiatry, 168,* 89–96.

Vaurio, O., Repo-Tiihonen, E., Kautiainen, H., & Tiihonen, J. (2018). Psychopathy and mortality. *Journal of Forensic Science, 63,* 474–477.

Vukasović, T., & Bratko, D. (2015). Heritability of personality: A meta-analysis of behavior genetic studies. *Psychological Bulletin, 141,* 769–785.

Wadsworth, M., Kuh, D., Richards, M., & Hardy, R. (2006). Cohort Profile: The 1946 National Birth Cohort (MRC National Survey of Health and Development). *International Journal of Epidemiology, 35,* 49–54.

Wafa, M. H., Viprey, M., Magaud, L., Haesebaert, J., Leaune, E., Poulet, E., Bied, C., & Schott, A-M. (2019). Identification of biopsychosocial factors predictive of post-traumatic stress disorder in patients admitted to the emergency department after a trauma (ISSUE): Protocol for a multicenter prospective study. *BMC Psychiatry, 19,* 163. https://doi.org/10.1186/s12888-019-2154-z

Wagner, A. C., Monson, C. M., & Hart, T. L. (2016). Understanding social factors in the context of trauma: Implications for measurement and intervention. *Journal of Aggression, Maltreatment & Trauma, 25,* 831–853.

Wampold, B. E. (2001). *The great psychotherapy debate: Models, methods, and findings.* Erlbaum Associates.

Wampold, B. E. (2019). A smorgasbord of PTSD treatments: What does this say about integration? *Journal of Psychotherapy Integration, 29,* 65–71.

Wampold, B. E., Imel, B. E., Laska, K. M., Benish, S., Miller, S. D., Flückiger, C., Del Re, A. C., Baardseth, T. P., & Budge, S. (2010). Determining what works in the treatment of PTSD. *Clinical Psychology Review, 30,* 923–933.

Weisberg, Y. J., Deyoung, C. G., & Hirsh, J. B. (2011). Gender differences in personality across the ten aspects of the Big Five. *Frontiers in Psychology, 2,* 178. https://doi.org/10.3389/fpsyg.2011.00178

Weiss, D. S., Marmar, C. R., Schlenger, W. E., Fairbank, J. A., Jordan, B. K., Hough, R. L., & Kulka, R. A. (1992). The prevalence of lifetime and partial post-traumatic stress disorder in Vietnam theater veterans. *Journal of Traumatic Stress, 5,* 365–372.

Weissman, M. M., Markowitz, J. C., & Klerman, G. L. (2000). *Comprehensive guide to interpersonal psychotherapy.* Basic Books.

Werner, E. E., & Smith, R. S. (1992). *Overcoming the odds: High-risk children from birth to adulthood.* Cornell University Press.

Wertz, J., Caspi, A., Ambler, A., Arseneault, L., Belsky, D. W., Danese, A., Fisher, H. L., Matthews, T., Richmond-Rakerd, L. S., & Moffitt, T. E. (2020). Borderline symptoms at age 12 signal risk for poor outcomes during the transition to adulthood: Findings from a genetically sensitive longitudinal cohort study. *Journal of the American Academy of Child and Adolescent Psychiatry, 59*(10), 1165–1177.

Widom, C. W. (1999). Posttraumatic stress disorder in abused and neglected children grown up. *American Journal of Psychiatry, 156,* 1223–1229.

Wiens, K., Bhattarai, A., Dores, A., Pedram, P., & Patten, S. (2020). Mental health among Canadian post-secondary students: A mental health crisis? *Canadian Journal of Psychiatry, 65,* 30–35.

Williams, F. M. K., Freydin, M., Mangino, M., Couvreur, S., Visconti, A., Bowyer, R. C. E., Le Roy, C. I., Falchi, M., Sudre, C., Davies, R., Hammond, D., Menni, C., Steves, C. J., & Spector, T. D. (2020). Self-reported symptoms of Covid-19 including symptoms most predictive of SARS-CoV-2 infection, are heritable. *Twin Research and Human Genetics, 23*(6), 316–321.

World Health Organization. (2019). *International Classification of Diseases* (11th ed.). WHO.

Yehuda, R. (Ed.). (1999). *Risk factors for posttraumatic stress disorder.* American Psychiatric Press.

Yehuda, R. (2002). Post-traumatic stress disorder. *New England Journal of Medicine, 346,* 108–114.

Yehuda, R., & Lehmer, A. (2018). Intergenerational transmission of trauma effects: Putative role of epigenetic mechanisms. *World Psychiatry, 17,* 243–257.

Yehuda, R., & McFarlane, A. C. (1995). Conflict between current knowledge about posttraumatic stress disorder and its original conceptual basis. *American Journal of Psychiatry, 152,* 1705–1713.

Young, A. (1995). *The harmony of illusions: Inventing post-traumatic stress disorder.* Princeton University Press.

Young, A., & Breslau, N. (2016). What is "PTSD"? The heterogeneity thesis. In D. E. Hinton & B. J. Good (Eds.), *Culture and PTSD: Trauma in global and historical perspective* (pp. 135–154). University of Pennsylvania Press.

Yuan, K., Gong, Y-M., Liu, L. Yan-Kun, S., Tian, S-S., Wang, Y-J., Zhong, Y., Zhang, A-Y., Su, S-Z., Liu, S-S., Zhang, Y-X., Lin, X., Shi, L., Yan, W., Fazel, S., Vitiello, M. V., Bryant, R. A., Zhou, X-Y., Ran, M-S., . . . Lu, L. (2021). Prevalence of posttraumatic stress disorder after infectious disease pandemics in the twenty-first century, including COVID-19: A meta-analysis and systematic review. *Molecular Psychiatry, 26*(9), 4982–4998.

Zanarini, M. C. (2000). Childhood experiences associated with the development of borderline personality disorder. *Psychiatric Clinics of North America, 23*, 89–101.

Zanarini, M. C. (2005). *Textbook of borderline personality disorder*. Taylor & Francis.

Zanarini, M. C., Frankenburg, F. R., Reich, D. B., Marino, M. F., Haynes, M. C., & Gunderson, J. G. (1999). Violence in the lives of adult borderline patients. *Journal of Nervous and Mental Disease, 187*(2), 65–71.

Zanarini, M. C., Temes, C. M., Magni, L. R., Fitzmaurice, G. M., Aguirre, B. A., & Goodman, M. (2017). Prevalence rates of borderline symptoms reported by adolescent inpatients with BPD, psychiatrically healthy adolescents and adult inpatients with BPD. *Personality and Mental Health, 11*, 150–156.

Zlotnick, C., Johnson, J., Kohn, R., Vicente, B., Rioseco, P., & Saldivia, S. (2006). Epidemiology of trauma, post-traumatic stress disorder (PTSD) and co-morbid disorders in Chile. *Psychological Medicine, 36*, 1523–1533.

Zweig-Frank, H., Paris, J., & Guzder, J. (1994). Psychological risk factors for dissociation in female patients with borderline and non-borderline personality disorders. *Journal of Personality Disorders, 8*, 203–209.

INDEX